PSYCHOTHERAPY IN THE AGE OF POLITICAL POLARIZATION

A Guide for Mental Health Professionals

William McCown and Linda Chamberlain

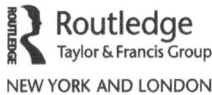

Routledge
Taylor & Francis Group

NEW YORK AND LONDON

Designed cover image: Getty Images

First published 2025
by Routledge
605 Third Avenue, New York, NY 10158

and by Routledge
4 Park Square, Milton Park, Abingdon, Oxon, OX14 4RN

Routledge is an imprint of the Taylor & Francis Group, an informa business

ISBN: 978-1-032-65119-4 (hbk)
ISBN: 978-1-032-65112-5 (pbk)
ISBN: 978-1-032-65121-7 (ebk)

DOI: 10.4324/9781032651217

Typeset in Times New Roman
by Newgen Publishing UK

PSYCHOTHERAPY IN THE AGE OF POLITICAL POLARIZATION

Psychotherapy in the Age of Political Polarization is a response to the challenge so many mental health professionals face: How do we best assist our clients who are suffering from the political polarization that is pervasive in our culture? This book explores how highly politicized interactions can often affect psychotherapy and counseling, and ways to combat the division.

The liberal/conservative division that exists in psychotherapy is discussed, and ways of overcoming these differences to work on a common goal in a therapeutic setting is of central importance. Useful case examples and vignettes are included to aid and mend divisions caused when encountering politically and ideologically challenging clients. Furthermore, the book explores how we've become so divided, the relevance of politics in therapy, the interface of political polarization with psychological disorders, and finally skills to aid mental health professionals in ethical practice.

This is an essential read for mental health professionals and students, including social workers, psychotherapists, counselors, and psychologists hoping to bridge the gap and reduce the negative impact of political polarization.

William McCown, PhD, is a licensed clinical psychologist and professor at the University of Louisiana Monroe, where he has taught for over 30 years and held various administrative roles. He earned his doctorate from Loyola University Chicago and completed a clinical internship at Tulane University Medical Center, specializing in both adult and child psychology. His clinical interests include gambling disorders, motivational problems, and neurodiversities. Much of his research has focused on measuring and treating chronic procrastination and exploring nonlinear systems in human behavior.

Linda Chamberlain, PsyD, is a licensed psychologist and professor (retired) with the Social and Human Services program at Pasco-Hernando State College in New Port Richey, Florida. She has worked as both an educator and clinician in the field of psychology and human services for 50 years. Dr. Chamberlain has authored and edited several books, including *Practicing Psychotherapy: Lessons on Helping Patients and Growing as a Professional* published in 2021 by Routledge/Taylor & Francis, and has been an invited speaker at local, national, and international conferences. She also serves as the co-moderator of the Mental Health Professionals Forum with Braver Angels.

"*Psychotherapy in the Age of Political Polarization: A Guide for Mental Health Professionals* is a timely must-read for mental health students and professionals seeking to better understand the contemporary political and social influences on the lives of our clients."

Zander Keig, *NASW, Social Worker of the Year (2020)*

"This book addresses a serious issue in the mental health field. Conservatives have a difficult time finding a therapist they can trust. In other contexts, therapists have come to understand that they must be knowledgeable and sensitive to the beliefs and values of their clients. It is time to recognize this is also true of political orientation."

Paul Norris, *LMFT, associate director, Braver Angels Debate Program*

"Politics, and the political strife that characterizes contemporary American society, inform clients' sense of identity, belongingness, and psychological safety. Our clients inevitably bring political issues to the consulting room, not merely as opinions, but as crucibles for defining their world-view and their sense of place and purpose in society. The inherent tension between the fundamental human need for interpersonal connection, versus the rampant and worsening alienation and fragmentation in the body politic, endangers well-being at all levels—family, neighborhood, community, and workplace. Drs. McCown and Chamberlain courageously take on a delicate task: bringing solid research perspectives to bear to illuminate an ethically sensitive and clinically meaningful approach to these issues, with the therapeutic mission and the well-being of the client always in the foreground. This is timely and valuable work, especially but not only for early career clinicians and those in training."

Jonathan Richard, *PsyD, clinical psychologist*

"William McCown and Linda Chamberlain brilliantly elucidate how the emotional and psychological impact of deep political divisions may become reflected within the therapy relationship. Demonstrating how political views are deeply rooted in people's identities and values, they further illustrate how disagreements can fracture the therapeutic alliance, create a breach of trust, or lead to irreparable treatment ruptures. McCown and Chamberlain enrich our understanding of the political divide by offering information and skills that mental health professionals can incorporate into their practices, including the importance of empathy, non-judgment, and communication skills, and fostering a deeper understanding of shared human experiences. The effects of extreme partisanship and its impact on treatment and relationships are certainly not taught to mental health professionals, who inevitably encounter this phenomenon in their practices. Skillfully, sensitively, and intentionally, McCown and Chamberlain guide clinicians to approach rather than avoid or fear issues of political partisanship in their work. *Psychotherapy in the Age of Political Polarization* is a great learning source for any mental health clinician."

Mary Lamia, *PhD, clinical psychologist, psychoanalyst, professor, author*

"The authors stress a fundamental truth: Human beings are more alike than they are unalike, and thus, all have the foundational need to be emotionally healthy. These authors know the 'social territory' and how to navigate the present terrain. They offer down-to-earth practical strategies on how to do just that. The case studies help readers to visualize the effectiveness of these strategies and further demonstrate the authors' collective expertise. A job well done!"

Pamela Higgins Saulsberry, *PhD, LCSW-BACS,*
Professor Emeritus of Social Work, University of Louisiana at Monroe

"Therapists can no longer afford to ignore the sequelae between race, gender, and politics particularly among those existing on the margins of American society (i.e., Blacks, Asians, women, children, LGBTQIA). Political polarization continues to negatively impact these groups at disproportionate rates on a local, state, and national scale. This book allows the reader(s) to engage in critical discourse about how these factors can inform their therapeutic practice and patient-counselor interactions. Each chapter offers the reader(s) how political polarization affects individuals, groups, and families across all human systems (e.g., micro, macro, and mezzo). I strongly recommend this book for practitioners concerned with learning practical ways and theoretical-based ways of achieving authentic communities with marginalized communities."

Raymond Adams, *PhD, MSW, MPH, associate professor,*
Morgan State University School of Social Work,
Editor-in-Chief of Journal of Social Work in Public Health

We dedicate this book to all who honor democracy by listening to, learning from, and working with those who challenge their views.

CONTENTS

Preface   *xi*
Acknowledgments   *xiv*

1 The Great Divide   1

2 Left and Right: Models of Liberal/Conservative
   Differences   15

3 Political to Partisan: How We Got Here   33

4 The Question of Liberal Bias in Mental Health
   Professionals   49

5 Politics Invades the Therapy Space   68

6 Empathy in Counseling the Politicized Client   83

7 Partisanship and Grief   102

8 Complex Disorders and Politics   116

9 Politics, Substance Abuse, and Addictive Behaviors   139

10 Working with Polarization in Relationships and Families   156

11 Depolarization, Training, and Support   173

12 Ethics and Advocacy   185

Appendix A: Political Orientation and Therapeutic Outcomes   *205*
Appendix B: Resources and Recommended Reading   *208*
Index   *215*

PREFACE

The ongoing division between people on the Left and the Right is unprecedented and accelerating worldwide. Linda and other "chaos theorists" might argue that this is an emergent phenomenon where small individual behaviors and attitudes interact, gradually forming larger and more dominant trends that are complex and often unpredictable. Yet recent events such as the war in Ukraine, the Gaza conflict, the 2024 US Presidential election, recent elections in Europe, and the rapid advances in AI, which have and will continue to foster disinformation, have only deepened this rift. This creates a truly alarming situation for everyone, except perhaps anarchists, as these forces amplify and potentially destabilize both public and private spheres.

Mental health services, in particular, are often delivered from a politically progressive stance, with many practitioners identifying as left-leaning or progressive.. Yet, in the United States, at least half of the population holds conservative views. These people often maintain deeply held beliefs that contrast sharply with the assumptions of many in the mental health profession, which is typically rooted in humanistic, science-based values. This disconnect can lead to tensions, as the values upheld by the profession may clash with those of conservative clients, leaving them feeling misunderstood or alienated in therapeutic settings.

This volume is not intended as a scholarly work but rather a scholarship-informed exploration of where we stand and what actions we might take. Its goal is to open up an important conversation about a critical issue that few are willing to address: the encroachment of politics into the therapy space. As political tensions increasingly affect therapeutic relationships, we find ourselves navigating new and uncertain ethical territory, often without basic tools for our ongoing tasks. To help illustrate these challenges, the volume includes vignettes and clinical histories, all of which are real but thoroughly anonymized to protect identities, with consent obtained for their use. Clinical narratives often convey the complexity of this issue more effectively than other methods.

We have endeavored to balance scholarship with accessibility, minimizing citations and references where appropriate. Readers may notice long passages with minimal citations, especially for what is now considered routine practice or common knowledge. Given the rapidly evolving nature of this topic, if we have missed your research or contribution, we humbly apologize. As the appendix shows, this volume is not focused on presenting new findings. Our ongoing inquiry in this area is discussed in relation to the rapidly growing and unpredictable condition that people across the political spectrum may be noticing.

Additionally, you may notice that we sometimes refer to mental health professionals as psychotherapists, clinicians, and counselors. For our purposes, there is no distinction between them, and we deeply appreciate the contributions of all mental health professionals in addressing these complex challenges. This book does not claim to offer definitive solutions but seeks to foster dialogue around this largely undiscussed and uncomfortable problem. We hope that all of us, regardless of our politics, professional affiliation, gender or orientation, geography, or nationality, will work to find a useful, humane solution.

William McCown

In the early months of 2022, following retirement from my faculty position at Pasco-Hernando State College, I was working at home providing telehealth psychotherapy and considering my next writing project. One of the phenomena that had caught my attention with therapy clients was the increase in anxiety, depression, and relationship problems related to politics and social issues. I was hearing more reports from clients of arguments with friends, neighbors, and family members about politics, high levels of distress about social policy issues, feeling worried about the future of the country, and a fear that things were coming apart in our ability to resolve the problems we faced. People were struggling to make choices about whether to have children, how to stay connected to people they loved but disagreed with, and whether to move to a place where they felt more comfortable and welcome politically.

In almost 50 years of practice as a psychotherapist, I was certainly familiar with working to help clients improve their relationships, effectively manage anxiety and depression, and cope with the challenges that we face in life. It was the connection of these familiar challenges with a factor that I hadn't really considered previously: politics. It made sense to me. I had my own struggles with the degree of distress and animosity that was entering conversations about political issues. The concern and anxiety that some of my clients felt, I felt too.

During this time, as I was experiencing an increase in mental health concerns related to political and social issues, I received a message from my colleague and writing partner, Dr. William (Bill) McCown. There had been a 25-year gap in our correspondence when he reached out to me with a proposal to write together again. Bill was also exploring the impact of political polarization on people's lives and well-being and wanted to write a book about the interface of politics and psychotherapy. We had co-authored other books on chaos theory in psychology and on problem gambling when our curiosity about those topics coincided in the past. Once again, we had both arrived at the same place regarding a compelling interest and desire to better understand the impact politics was having on our profession and those we served.

This book has been a wonderful opportunity to connect again with Bill for which I am deeply grateful. The renewal of our friendship and partnership as writers has brought me great joy. I hope that our collaboration will be a useful resource for other mental health professionals who are being confronted with the impact of politics on themselves and those they serve. This is a topic that deserves more attention and research so that we, as mental health professionals, can better understand and help others.

Linda Chamberlain

ACKNOWLEDGMENTS

My thanks for the support and encouragement of so many colleagues; Dr. Jon Richard, Paul Norris, Mary Beth Stibbins, and members of the Braver Angels Mental Health Professionals Forum, Cheryl Dolinger Brown, Dr. Andrew Hartz of the Open Therapy Institute, Dr. Bill Doherty, therapists with Better Help who shared their experiences working with clients impacted by political polarization, and many others who shared information and resources in support of this book. I'm equally grateful to those clients who helped me understand the importance of learning to work with political diversity. Thank you for your patience as I learned along with you how to better communicate about these issues.

I appreciate friends and family who helped me stay focused and provided much needed encouragement, and occasional very welcome distractions, during the writing process. Thanks to Dr. Pat Maher, Jessica Welsh, Patty and Steve MacLauchlain, Bob Crow, Barbara Ravis, Paloma Sparrowhawk, and many others.

Most importantly, thank you to my partner and a terrific writer himself, Jeff McBee. I'm grateful for your understanding when I needed to spend days writing and reading materials for this book, for being so helpful with chores that needed attention when I was in the middle of working, and for the love and support you have always shared with me. You're the best.

Linda Chamberlain

I am deeply grateful to everyone who opened up, taking the time to talk with us: clinicians, counselors, clients, and their families.

I owe special thanks to Dr. Joanne Yaffe, Professor Emeritus, University of Utah, for her constant insight and joyous surprises and to Dr. Mary Lamia, psychoanalyst and affect theorist, who was so personally kind and helpful throughout this time in my life.

Some of the ideas for this book owe much to discussions with the late Dr. Scott Lilienfeld, the generous, brilliant psychologist who was very much attuned to the way that cultural wars influence psychological treatment. His passing was a profound loss to all mental health professionals. I also wish to honor the late Dr. Greg Stolcis, who foresaw the liberal/conservative division in therapy 30 years ago and worked to stop it. I am also very grateful to the late Dr. Sean Austin, a longtime mentor whose guidance has been invaluable.

I am so very thankful to colleagues on all sides of the political spectrum, most of whom want to remain anonymous. But on the right, these include Dr. Julie Nelson, past president of the Louisiana Psychological Association, and Dr. Ross Keiser; and leaning more left, the late Gary Thompson, Dr. Jack and the late Linda Palmer, and Dr. Wendel Ray. I also appreciate the support of so many friends through the years: Drs. Burt Ashworth, John "Jodey" Edwards, Joseph Ferrari, Rob Hanser, Joe McGahan, Janelle McDaniel, Rick Stevens, John Sutherlin, Myrna Shure, Jan Sutton, Scott Shelby, Seth Tackett, Scott Zentner, and many more kind, inquisitive people.

Melba and Jimmy Dulaney and their amazing family mean more to me than I deserve. I can never be grateful enough.

Most of all, I am profoundly thankful to Wendy, Ivy, Gavin, and Quinton for their love, patience, and unwavering support. You have taught me what I never learned earlier and I hope I've been worth the hassle.

William McCown

1

THE GREAT DIVIDE

An Overview of the Liberal/Conservative Gap in Society, Counseling, and Psychotherapy

> I see clients asking me how I voted, who I supported, my views on immigration, abortion, even prayer in school. And I feel unprepared. I also feel a bit resentful. One client told me she had 'burned up,' and that was her term, the Internet, to determine if I was liberal. I entered this profession to be a healer. I didn't enter it to watch my politics. So I just don't say anything. Ever.
>
> (Psychologist in a Northeast state)

> How I feel about politics is a big part of my life. The fact that I could tell my counselor everything, horrible thought really, except not at all about how I voted was just creepy to me. It is not honest.
>
> (A client in Western USA)

The United States, Great Britain, Canada, many parts of Europe, and elsewhere are experiencing remarkable increases in political divisiveness (Jost, Baldassarri, & Druckman, 2022; McCarty, 2019). Although the reasons for this are controversial, somewhat uncertain, and likely very complex, what is clear to most people is that political rancor has substantially increased in recent years. The levels of divisiveness, which spills over to many aspects of life, should profoundly matter to mental health professionals. With the increased polarization that society is experiencing, this trend appears likely to continue.

If you are a therapist, counselor, mental health professional, or mental health professional-in-training, you may have already experienced the side

DOI: 10.4324/9781032651217-1

effects of this polarization. There is already a high probability that you have encountered a client or patient who wants to know about your politics, religion, and personal beliefs. A few years ago, these topics were usually considered taboo. Now, however, we would be surprised if you hadn't been directly queried or scrutinized closely on social media for clues regarding how you vote and your opinions on gun control, immigration, abortion, overseas wars, or other current, "hot topic" issues.

Mental health professionals are usually well-trained to deflect personal questions and separate their feelings from their clients'. Unfortunately, our training has rarely prepared us for the politicization too often occurring in "the therapy space" (Chamberlain, 2021), the once untouchable process of therapy. As part of our classwork, training, and supervision, we learn procedures to deal with extreme crises and people with a variety of intense behavior disorders. We have not, however, been taught to pay sufficient attention to addressing the needs of increasingly partisan clients. In this book, we offer guidelines about responding to questions from clients regarding our worldviews and where we stand on social and political issues. No one teaches us to handle our thoughts and emotions when clients present worldviews that collide with ours and seem offensive or wrong to us. Moreover, we have little training on what to do if a client espouses ideologies that we percieve are not only harmful and hurtful but also potentially dangerous.

Until recently, remarkably little attention has been paid to how political divisions affect academic mental health disciplines or the practice of providing mental health services (Frisby, Redding, O'Donohue, & Lilienfeld, 2023). Researchers and therapists, however, are beginning to note that politics too often impinge on the therapy process. A study by Solomonov and Barber (2019) illustrated how a therapist's self-disclosure of political feelings affects the therapeutic alliance. According to their data, almost 87% of therapists surveyed said they discussed politics during sessions, and 63% reported political self-disclosure. Those who perceived political similarity with patients were likelier to have political discussions and a higher self-rated therapeutic alliance. At the time of their study, more left-leaning psychotherapists reported their clients who supported Hillary Clinton showed increased political tensions and more negative emotions following the 2016 presidential election, with the opposite for Donald Trump supporters. They concluded that politics play a crucial role in therapeutic processes, whether therapists and counselors choose to admit this or not. As is true with other aspects of a client's life, like sexual orientation or religion, perceived similarity with a therapist may affect decisions to self-disclose and the quality of the therapeutic alliance.

In today's volatile political landscape, many counselors and therapists now encounter clients who feel threatened or cued by therapists' political orientations. Not surprisingly, more and more mental health professionals report being uncomfortable with these emerging areas. Yet mental health professionals have rarely discussed this issue and suggested directions toward workable solutions. At a minimum, the purpose of this book is to begin the discussion so mental health professionals can examine our shared profession in order to have conversations about effective and ethical clinical approaches to political issues that arise in treatment. Later chapters will discuss how the liberal/conservative divide affects factors associated with psychotherapeutic success. We will also present case studies that we hope may suggest potentially valuable techniques for a range of partisan clients, including those on the more toxic extremes. However, our primary purpose is to raise awareness that counseling and psychotherapy cannot live in an isolative bubble, ignoring the political realities of the outside world while continuing to treat clients with political views that are vastly different from many of their providers.

Left and Right: Who Gets Treated and How?

Another argument of this book is that many people who lean in the direction of conservative do not feel comfortable in counseling or psychotherapy. Too often, they do not trust practitioners whom they think may be too progressive to understand their values and lifestyles. Furthermore, some politically liberal therapists do not feel comfortable treating conservative clients. This can be an onerous burden because most therapists are at least politically moderate or moderately liberal. The reality is that many clients are more conservative than practitioners attempting to help them. Consequently, many therapists and clients may feel awkward with each other and even mutually distrustful. This can strain a therapeutic alliance and undermine treatment. A similar effect occurs when conservative therapists treat very liberal clients. This is less common, however, since most therapists are at least politically moderate, and many lean more liberal, as we shall argue in Chapter 4.

Curiously, current graduate training programs have neglected the vast cultural differences between people on the Right and Left and how that might affect therapy and counseling. In contemporary graduate school, almost all therapists-in-training now have courses in multicultural intervention. Students strive to put aside preconceptions and view diverse cultures with a lens of equity, nonjudgmental understanding, and sincere tolerance or appreciation. Oddly, this lens omits a central, perhaps overpowering cultural division in the United States and increasingly elsewhere, which is political. Almost every practitioner agrees that no one should graduate from a reputable mental health program without realizing that basic cultural competence and tolerance are essential for effective, ethical clinical practice (Vasquez & Johnson, 2022). Yet we graduate practitioners who are not taught to respect and tolerate the diverse political values that people embody.

Despite these frequent mismatches, very little research has been done on how severe the liberal/conservative divide in therapy might well be. This is somewhat surprising. After all, political affiliation is another cultural influence we all bring to the therapy session, whether we're the therapist or the client (Farber, 2018). This is well understood in other areas, including gender, race and ethnicity, and religion. Notably, there are over 57,000 articles, posters, professional presentations, book chapters, and books on gender differences and multicultural facets in psychotherapy. This attention is undoubtedly appropriate, since it has helped people become better, more sensitive, and more equitable therapists, and we certainly support this training. However, less than one-quarter of similar sources address the liberal and conservative split in therapy. Most are theoretical or case studies rather than research-based findings.

Regardless, there is emerging evidence that more liberal counselors view the therapeutic process differently than conservatives. For example, Norton and Tan (2019) examined the role of political ideologies in a large group of licensed mental health counselors and its relation to counseling theories used in clinical practice. Not surprisingly, they found that the majority of counselors identified as politically liberal. Self-identification as conservative predicted a preference for cognitive behavioral therapies. Self-identified liberals showed a preference for psychodynamic theory.

Politics and Personal Identity

There is a more subtle reason that mental health professionals need to learn to be tolerant of all political orientations. Therapy is often where people turn to develop or validate their life narratives. Developing a political identity is essential to many people's identities and life stories. Yet many therapists do not seem to realize this. They may be comfortable with clients as they discuss a variety of intimate topics: sexuality, abuse, deep secrets, achievements, addictions, successes, and hidden shame. Yet they may be very uncomfortable discussing politics as part of a person's history, dreams, and visions. Political discussions are a part of life. As our society continues to fracture, they will become increasingly common and even more critical in the therapy relationship. For example, following the Supreme Court's decision to overturn Roe v. Wade and take away a woman's right to choose abortion, several clients of one of the authors sought therapy because of the ruling's very personal impact on them and their identity. These discussions required an understanding and discussion of politics that some practitioners might avoid.

Unlike many other developmental tasks, there is no expected period for creating a personal political orientation. People have no socially prescribed timeframe to explore and develop their political feelings. Unlike career identification and development, leaving home, developing a romantic or sexual identity, or adopting a religious affiliation, there is no socially recognized normative period when people can explore available political options and see what fits best with their core beliefs. People often lock into their families' and peers' political worldviews. They may discuss these in therapy at any point in their life cycles, just as they might have different relationship challenges or trouble with family members at different times in their lives.

Developing a political worldview may be a gradual or even recurrent process over the lifespan. This is different from an abruptly discontinuous identity change. Abrupt identity changes, whether religious, vocational, familial, or even more intimate, can often be disruptive, stressful, and costly. The process of political polarization is a disruptive change, as therapists intuitively seem to realize, though one that is increasingly common. Political polarization sometimes occurs when more moderate people swing abruptly in a more extreme direction, often due to economic downturns or personal tragedies. Stress or catastrophic events can also contribute to polarizing political views. The polarization, in turn, becomes stress. This is more likely when political affiliation changes quickly, firmly, or disruptively in the life cycle.

Chamberlain (2021) and many other authors have noted that culture is intimately tied to how people think of and disclose their constructed selves. People discussing their political orientations highlight their social and personal identities. Yet, by implication, people often contrast themselves with those with opposite views. The process can become toxic when disagreement moves toward disparaging then dehumanizing those who disagree. This is common among highly polarized people. For example, a liberal activist might define their politics as "Pro-marginalized people, pro-feminist, environmental, and pro-animal rights." In other words, "I support the welfare of others." This implies that those on the other side lack these very humane interests and virtues. They may also espouse the perspective that "I am anti-fascist, antiracist, anti-big Pharma, and anti-destruction of the earth" and believe that those on the conservative side of the spectrum embrace the opposite viewpoint. It is often difficult for people on the political extreme to think that those on the other end of the spectrum are, in most respects, fundamentally good people like themselves.

Good people may differ regarding what moral dimension they attend to, skewing their judgments (Haidt & Graham, 2007). Conservatives, like liberals, often assert their identity by noting specific values. These tend to be phrased equally forcefully and positively, often in terms of human interests. For example, a conservative person might say, "I am pro-job, pro-freedom, pro-growth, and I support individual and family responsibility." Their definitions of those with more liberal values might include "They are pro-big government, soft on crime, and for radicals teaching children in our schools." Not very good people, are they?

Divisive political rhetoric has now become so ubiquitous that few people, including therapists, feel much meaningful dialogue is possible. However, dialogue is necessary for the development of both compromise and a life narrative. Without dialogue, people define their thinking in ways that discount those who disagree. Both the politically oriented media and local politics are now rewarding a brasher, ruder interaction with little regard for the dignity of the opposition (Ferguson, 2023). Often, more polarized people disregard "Truth" in pursuit of higher goals. For them, it is appropriate to espouse a "noble lie" to defend the "greater good." Only the political cause matters and any action to meet this goal is reasonable. Soon, the other side embodies a variety of evils that are projected onto them. Single issues and other forms of intense politics have created a psychodynamic "splitting" situation. "We are good. They are bad." Furthermore, thinking becomes very emotional, characterized by absolute, black-and-white dichotomous choices characterized by accusations.

Some counselors or therapists believe that symptoms of emotionality and dichotomous thinking exhibited by politically extreme people are not too different from those displayed by people with Borderline Personality Disorder. They may also apply this description to society, commenting on how factions are split by hostility. While diagnostic metaphors applied to society are simply heuristics and should not be taken too literally, they may sometimes be helpful. It is as if numerous political communities are using borderline defenses, splitting the "good" and the "bad," vigorously reacting to parts of themselves that they do not want to accept. Groups have always done this, but the frequency and rancor are startling and unsettling. At times, it may be pathological and dominate specific individuals' thoughts.

In addition to an angry impulsivity and splitting, a hallmark of borderline symptoms is a fluctuating sense of identity. For some people, perhaps extreme political beliefs are a self-treatment for a lack of a coherent self. Adopting a political affiliation can give people a profound, convincing, all-consuming identity. In the extreme, this identity can become intertwined with a single political issue, where a sole idea dominates someone's political thought and interest. Often, these people seem angry and aggrieved but certainly focused and passionate. In essence, they become both highly motivated and, often to others, increasingly toxic. In Chapter 8, we will further discuss how politically radicalized citizens may sometimes be so toxic that they resemble people with Borderline Disorder and those with other forms of severe psychopathologies.

Regardless of how far we take this borderline analogy, the black-and-white thinking associated with mono-issue politics has drastic interpersonal consequences. It typically takes emotional effort to be discreet, caring, and compassionate. Some people see these behaviors as unnecessary for those who are not like themselves. They may believe that they are on the "correct side," and the opposition simply is not. If you feel something deeply, those who do not think as you do are probably various shades of "bad" or "wrong" and may not deserve to be treated with the decency and compassion that is extended to like-minded people.

The world soon becomes seen through a lens of "us against them." Events like mass shootings in the United States are seen through a filtered perspective of evil and good, black and white. People on the Right see these as evidence that America has become too soft on crime and that armed citizens need to increase their vigilance. People on the Left see the same occurrences and agree with their significance, but they radically disagree with their interpretation. They believe these events are due to the availability of guns and the viciousness of contemporary culture, poverty, and a legacy of complex problems. Two viewpoints look at the same event and have diametrically opposite solutions. It is no wonder that we see others as the enemy of reason. And somehow, too often, clinicians and counselors do not understand that reasonable people can view events differently without being evil or ignorant.

False Consensus and Partisan Mindsets

There are many reasons that counselors and clinicians fail to understand how politics may be intruding on the therapeutic space. Some of these are rooted in our human nature. The false consensus effect is a cognitive bias that causes people to overestimate the degree to which their beliefs, opinions, preferences, values, and habits are typical of others (Ross, Greene, & House, 1977). This well-known social psychological effect makes people assume that most people are thinking similarly to themselves, especially in a group of like-minded individuals. For example, heavy drinkers normalize their drinking by hanging out with other problem drinkers, as do drug users or heavy gamblers. "We all do it," they reason, clear examples of overestimations from false consensus.

Clinicians often point out that their clients succumb to this effect. For example, a highly religious, somewhat eccentric-believing person may think their beliefs are within the mainstream when they clearly are not. As mental health professionals, we may sincerely, if gingerly, comment that most other people do not believe that the world will end in the next couple of months because of the advent of a newly prophesized Anti-Christ. Even though people in that person's small cult might firmly endorse it and affirm it to each other daily, this belief is outside of the mainstream. The belief was derived and strengthened from a false consensus. However, we may also miss the fact that our clients do not hold the same political beliefs that we have, partly because our own beliefs may be based on consensus from our own limited groups.

The false consensus effect leads to underestimating the general population's diversity of opinions, beliefs, and behaviors. It arises partly from limited exposure to various perspectives, especially in more homogenous social circles.

It also causes us to overgeneralize our life experiences to others who are different. For example, a conservative college president who grew up in poverty believes that just about everyone can follow her successful path and that society should design policies to encourage the path that worked to bring her out of her impoverishment. There might be no proof that what she did was scalable beyond her own life experiences. However, it is often human nature to believe that "what worked for my friends and me" will work for everyone else. This person might embark on a life quest to get people to emulate her specific path, not realizing that her life journey does not necessarily apply to others.

In politics, this type of thinking can result in people believing that their own experiences are the general roadmap for every other citizen. It works equally deceptively in counseling and therapy. The therapist may think, "If this client just had my values, they wouldn't be in this mess." When that happens, the therapist or counselor may become less empathetic, less genuine, less open, more judgmental, and more apt to focus on their own feelings instead of those of the client.

False consensus effects are partly due to cognitive heuristics, which are mental shortcuts that simplify decision-making. Assuming others are like us simplifies the complex task of understanding different people. It is also an element of wishing to conform to what is socially desirable or normative. By believing that one's opinions are widely shared, one can feel more confident and secure in one's views. Put simply, it is a very human, if irrational, response to complex social situations. However, it is not necessarily helpful in counseling or therapy.

The false consensus effect is not just a quirky error in our thinking. It is a fundamental aspect of how we relate to the social world (Greene, 2013). It shows how deeply our perspectives and experiences color our perception of the "average" or "typical" person. This bias can comfort and deceive us, leading to misunderstandings and conflicts. Yet, it also represents our natural tendency to seek connection and common ground with others. Just like in art, where perspective is everything, in psychology, our view of the social landscape is often painted with broad strokes of our own experiences and beliefs. This affects our clients, especially when it occurs without our awareness.

There are several other reasons why mental health professionals may be failing large numbers of clients. Beyond the tendency to look primarily at our own experiences and those of our group, therapists may form stereotypes about political discussions because they respond to an extreme subgroup of clients. Therapists may have exaggerated fears based on their experiences with complex or exceptional clients who present themselves as very partisan, even extremists. This aligns with extensive literature regarding how we form stereotypes and use heuristics or mental shortcuts. Therapists and counselors respond positively and negatively to media stereotypes and influences like everyone else. Therapists often believe highly opinionated clients are the most troublesome ones they can encounter, and they may have little training to help them interact effectively. They treat these stereotypes with fear rather than compassion.

Most liberals and conservatives attempt to maintain some distance between their political identities and other aspects of their lives. Even those who are not politically moderate can practice interpersonal moderation. There seems, however, to be an increasing number of what Eric Hoffer (1951/2002) calls "True Believers." These are people who have become transfixed by political or social mass movements and extreme ideas or baseless theories. People in any conceivable area of the political spectrum who embrace "alternative facts," conspiracy theories, and beliefs not grounded in evidence or reality can become profoundly dangerous in the hands of a charismatic leader. People fitting this description seem to be the clients that therapists are most wary of and respond to stereotypically. The stereotype that they trigger may generalize to all clients with highly partisan beliefs.

> I don't do well with conservativism. They trigger feelings in me about Nazis. That is my issue, but most of the time, I struggle to be aware of it.
>
> *(A counselor from the west coast)*

Sometimes, the most triggering people are those with a *highly partisan mindset.* Chamberlain (2021) describes addiction as a misplaced search for happiness. Similarly, extreme political views can be seen as a misplaced search for safety, justice, and community. In this process, political or ideological beliefs become a person's primary way of interacting with their environment. Extremists, whether Left or Right, tend to be similar. They may have different beliefs, but their cognitive processes and social behavior are often remarkably uniform. They share a *partisan mindset* when their identity increasingly intertwines with their politics. Usually, they use their identity to try to control aspects of the environment that they believe are dangerous or otherwise threatening.

Beyond the partisan mindset, a *partisan identity* involves developing a personality that is based on a comparison to dichotomous opposites (Rychlak, 2003). The more forcefully a belief is held, the firmer the certainty that the opposite is false. As Rychlak argued, we tend to think about new concepts or constructs in a binary, opposing fashion; this observation is not new and was made in classic research studies by George Kelly (Sechrest, 1963) and many others. We classify what we have learned logically by what it is but simultaneously by what it is not. Rychlak (2003) calls this "logical learning theory," the almost Zen-like idea that to know something is also to know something of its opposite. Whether this is always true is controversial. But when incorporating a new, over-arching belief, we generally reclassify our previous categories into more manageable extremes. Strong opinions result in strong opposites with little room for shades of subtlety.

In Chapter 3, we will argue that this type of opponent process is why the direct confrontation of irrational beliefs in therapy is often counterproductive.

History proves that a highly partisan mindset, either on the Left or Right, is potentially quite dangerous to those who do not endorse it. These beliefs can become toxic when they bias their adherents to become keenly aware of every "unfair critique" from the other side and simultaneously make them oblivious to their own side's errors or misdeeds (Novoa et al., 2023). People with highly partisan mindsets share many similarities, as we'll examine further in Chapter 3. One of the most important similarities is the tendency to devalue logic and evidence. The highly partisan mind represents a crystallization of what has been called "felt knowledge" (Gollwitzer et al., 2023). This differs from opinion and belief. Felt knowledge, or excessive subjective certainty, involves more mental rigidity than mere belief. It is less founded on one's experience and factual reality and more on emotional reactions. People on the extremes of the Left and Right "know" something is true, regardless of the weight of the evidence *and regardless of whether others can know it.* Although we saw this with many conservatives regarding the 2020 Presidential outcome, extreme liberal people also have their share of subjective truths that they believe are unassailable.

In Chapter 3, we argue that the toxic extremes of a partisan mindset are developed partly through *discordant knowing* (Gollwitzer et al., 2023). In discordant knowing, counterfactual statements have been found to reiterate core beliefs. In other words, disconfirmation in therapy or counseling may increase a partisan mindset. Tell someone something that they disagree with, and they will not only contradict you, but they will also come to believe it even more. Therapists can drive people toward more extreme beliefs merely by arguing or persuading them to abandon their more bizarre cognitions. The more you argue, the more they believe.

The following examples of client statements indicate that some counselors and therapists inadvertently further polarize their clients' views.

> I told my therapist the same thing I told my partner. I don't care how much you want to disagree with me about politics. You can argue all you want. It just makes me realize that I am right. No, I mean to say 'Correct.' Nothing about the way I think is right-wing voodoo … And if you are planning to contradict me, I will drill my spiked heels even deeper into the ground. The more you argue with me, the more I know I am right.
>
> *(Liberal female client, age 29)*

> My counselor's okay. She helps with my depression. But she tries to get me to give up my 2nd Amendment rights (right to own firearms in the US Constitution). Strange, isn't it? I tell her I'm depressed but I won't hurt

myself so please be quiet about my gun rights. No danger here. All this liberal agenda. You just make me want to buy another gun. Pretty soon she will be lecturing me about why I need an electric car.

(Conservative male, age 50+)

Overview of This Book

Our goal with this volume is to increase the awareness of practitioners working in our contemporary, fractured society. We must become aware that a problem exists before we can solve it. The first step in providing therapy in a multiculturally competent manner is awareness of a potential problem. We believe that this will allow counselors and therapists the ability, and perhaps the courage to assess and address their own political biases, assumptions, and misperceptions. Clients across the political spectrum deserve the same respect, acceptance, and consideration that are integral parts of being a culturally competent therapist.

The book will explore a variety of different factors regarding politics in the therapy space, from information on the dynamics that influence political persuasions to resources for depolarization. The following is an introduction to the topics that will be addressed.

Chapter 2 discusses how people form mental models of liberals and conservatives. We will attempt to illustrate various ways of classifying people according to their political interests and persuasions. By realizing this, we become less subjected to stereotyping. We further discuss whether there is any evidence for genuine differences between people on the left and the right and, if so, whether these differences genuinely matter as much as we assume.

Chapter 3 explores how society and our clients have become increasingly fractured. The chapter addresses the myth that the split is confined to one country or is due to one particular person or political party. It outlines how society made the long journey to the chronic disagreements that we are facing now. This is mirrored in the struggles that many of our clients' face, from being politically interested and motivated to being highly partisan and identifying with their own, sometimes bizarre beliefs to the exclusion of all else.

Chapter 4 highlights that many behavioral health providers lean in a liberal direction, although certainly with many exceptions. Clients, though, come from a variety of political positions. If we ignore the potential differences between the worldviews of our clients and ourselves, we may well impose our values and worldviews on clients without their consent. This is unethical, irresponsible, ineffective, and insensitive.

Chapter 5 examines some of the primary ways politics has entered the process of counseling and therapy, "the therapy space," and some helpful approaches. It is based on suggestions from practitioners who work with politically diverse clients.

Chapter 6 focuses on the importance and practice of empathy when working with political issues. Drawing on the experience of successful clinicians, this chapter explores various strategies and techniques that counselors can employ when working with highly politicized clients.

Chapter 7 looks at grief and loss in working with those impacted by political polarization. In a turbulent political climate, grief can become entangled with partisan beliefs and behaviors. This chapter explores the intersection of grief, group identity, political extremism, and polarization. We discuss how grief can also make people more vulnerable to extremist influences and how partisan conflict can be a source of loss and emotional pain.

Chapter 8 discusses how some psychological disorders can be impediments to counseling politicized clients. Specifically, it addresses bipolar disorders, personality disorders, paranoia, anger, distrust, and hostility. The chapter emphasizes that it is too easy to mistake political partisanship for mood, thought, or personality disorders. Primary psychiatric disorders must be treated and never ignored, regardless of the client's political views.

Chapter 9 highlights addiction and substance abuse and its relationship to politics. People on both the Left and the Right experience addictions and develop addictive behaviors. However, their stigma and responses are often different. Moreover, addictions can sometimes be used to mask mental disorders or family tensions, making the counselor or therapist's job even more difficult.

Chapter 10 considers a critical aspect of the political divide: the effect on couples and families. It is common for politics to interfere with family functioning, and this chapter has suggestions regarding working with political divisions in relationships. It is necessary to cope with genuine political grief and to move on to live, work, and sometimes even to love. We'll examine how political divisiveness impacts relationships from dating, to couples, parent-child dynamics, and extended families.

Chapter 11 discusses more advanced depolarization training for clinicians and the need for ongoing professional education and support. For some clients who are more deeply, irrationally politicized, more complex therapy may be necessary. Toxic political involvement can become all-consuming, threatening an individual's friendships, family ties, and perhaps their livelihood. This chapter also recognizes the importance of seeking advanced training and on-going supervision when working with polarized clients and their families.

Chapter 12 is an introduction to critical issues in ethics and advocacy for mental health professionals in today's highly politicized world. Ethical codes across mental health disciplines share a similar foundation. At their core, ethical principles within these fields emphasize beneficence (doing good), non-maleficence (avoiding harm), respect for client autonomy (their right to make choices), justice (providing fair and equitable treatment), and fidelity (honoring trust and responsibilities within the professional relationship). This chapter also invites mental health professionals to consider advocacy and roles beyond the therapy space. Some practitioners may consider taking on a more public role as a "citizen therapist" who acts as an advocate for societal change to mitigate polarization and divisiveness in our communities and country.

Summary

One of the primary objectives of this book is to promote a more impartial approach when working with clients who hold strong political views, whether they align with the right or the left. Maintaining a traditional stance of neutrality has become increasingly complex and challenging for practitioners in the helping professions. The purpose of this volume is not to teach people to alter an individual's political orientation, whether they lean right or left. That is both unethical and likely impossible. Nothing in this book suggests that either the left or the right has a monopoly on morality, intelligence, ethics, and values.

We acknowledge the importance of every individual's voice and believe that no respectful person should be excluded from meaningful dialogue. We are cognizant that change can be unsettling, and we recognize the need for people to be heard. Blanket intolerance toward others' views and suppressing voices on either side is detrimental to an open society. While we may find certain aspects of free speech highly offensive at times, and its content may even infuriate us, we must acknowledge that it represents a *possible* dialogue. As counselors or therapists, we can assist individuals in developing critical thinking skills and incorporating processes that foster the ability for more effective interchange, increased tolerance, and the ability to seek reasoned compromise. Ultimately, the choice rests with the clients. We cannot exclude them from the conversation or employ tactics of intolerance, whether they are partisans or extremists on the left or the right.

References

Chamberlain, L. (2021). *Practicing psychotherapy: Lessons on helping patients and growing as a professional.* New York: Routledge.

Farber, B. A. (2018). 'Clowns to the left of me, jokers to the right': Politics and psychotherapy, 2018. *Journal of Clinical Psychology, 74*(5), 714–721. https://doi.org/10.1002/jclp.22600

Ferguson, C. J. (2023). One psychologist's reasons for resigning from the American Psychological Association. In: Frisby, C. L., Redding, R. E., O'Donohue, W. T., & Lilienfeld, S. O. (Eds.), *Ideological and political bias in psychology.* Cham: Springer. https://doi.org/10.1007/978-3-031-29148-7_12

Frisby, C. L., Redding, R. E., O'Donohue, W. T. & Lilienfeld, S. O. (Eds.) (2023). *Ideological and political bias in psychology: Nature, scope and solutions.* Cham, Switzerland: Springer.

Gollwitzer, M., Prager, J., Altenmuller, M. S. & Zein, R .A. (2023). *Psychology Learning & Teaching*, *22*(3), 245–250.

Greene, J. (2013). *Moral tribes: Emotion, reason, and the gap between us and them.* Penguin Press.

Haidt, J., & Graham, J. (2007). When morality opposes justice: Conservatives have moral intuitions that liberals may not recognize. *Social Justice Research*, *20*(1), 19.

Jost, J. T., Baldassarri, D. S. & Druckman, J. N (August 2022). Cognitive–motivational mechanisms of political polarization in social-communicative contexts. *Nature Reviews Psychology*, *1*(1010), 560–576.

McCarty, N. (2019). *Polarization: What everyone needs to know*. London: Oxford Press. http://dx.doi.org/10.1093/wentk/9780190867782.001.0001

Norton, A. L., & Tan, T. X. (2019). The relationship between licensed mental health counselors' political ideology and counseling theory preference. *American Journal of Orthopsychiatry*, *89*(1), 86–93. https://doi.org/10.1007/s11211-

Novoa, G., Echelbarger, M., Gelman, A. & Gelman, S. A. (2023). Generically partisan: Polarization in political communication. *Proceedings of the National Academy of Sciences of the United States of America*, *120*(47), 1–17. https://doi.org/10.1073/pnas.2309361120

Rychlak, J. F. (2003). Personality theorizing as describing individuals or collectives. In J. F. Rychlak, *The human image in postmodern America* (pp. 17–31). American Psychological Association. https://doi.org/10.1037/10565-002

Sechrest, L. (1963). The psychology of personal constructs: George Kelly. In J. M. Wepman & R. W. Heine (Eds.), *Concepts of personality* (pp. 206–233). Aldine Publishing Co. https://doi.org/10.1037/11175-008

Solomonov, N. & Barber, J. P. (2019). Conducting psychotherapy in the Trump era: Therapists' perspectives on political self-disclosure, the therapeutic alliance, and politics in the therapy room. *Journal of Clinical Psychology*, *75*, 1508–1518. https://doi.org/10.1002/jclp.22801

Vasquez, M. J. T., & Johnson, J. D. (2022). Multicultural therapy: A practice imperative. Washington, DC: American Psychological Association. https://doi.org/10.1037/0000279-000

2

LEFT AND RIGHT

Models of Liberal/Conservative Differences

Models of the Left/Right Divide

So far, we have referred to people on the political Left and the Right, liberals and conservatives, as if everyone agrees on their characteristics. This is simply common sense, or so it seems. Everyone believes that they know how to characterize political opinions since we all have our own. Many things about our worldview may seem intuitive but are more complex, obscure, and ultimately more profound than our assumptions tell us. Stereotypes are never entirely correct, and often, they are substantially wrong. Sometimes, they result in highly biased thinking with profoundly damaging consequences, particularly in psychotherapy.

Attempting to get beyond common social stereotypes, behavioral scientists have long debated what, if any, specific attitudes and opinions define people on the Left and the Right. Still, many researchers argue that there is no clear consensus. One reason for the apparent confusion is that attitudes may relate to distinct cultures and periods rather than be as universal as we assume. For example, in contemporary Saudi Arabia, someone labeled as a political liberal may advocate for women to be allowed to drive a motor vehicle, which is hardly disturbing to most conservative people in Sweden or Mexico. As the well-known personality theorist Raymond Cattell noted long ago, looking beyond surface traits, even the ones that seem obvious, is usually necessary to find more useful causal models (Cattell & Kline, 1977).

There are many different models of how to classify liberals and conservatives. None are complete, nor should they claim to be unfailingly accurate. Models are heuristic, meaning that they reflect a picture of reality. The model is not

DOI: 10.4324/9781032651217-2

necessarily reality, any more than a map is the actual territory. Models are helpful when they assist us in organizing our thinking and making accurate predictions. Like maps, they are valuable if they help us find what we need. They are less useful when they interfere with understanding reality. Interference can occur when we insist that our model is reality rather than our construction of it.

Implicit Models: Us Against Them

Models may be personal and implicit or more formal and generalized. Although we do not usually realize it, we all make implicit models of people's politics. Implicit models are informal, internal representations people develop through experience to understand and interact with the world (Payne & Cameron, 2013). These models are based on associations, intuitions, and accumulated knowledge. Implicit models are not precisely defined and often operate primarily outside of conscious awareness. Implicit models are typically limited in scope and apply mainly to familiar situations (Chamberlain, 2021).

Implicit models allow us to form rapid judgments and guide us on how to act. For instance, when we interact with a stranger, our implicit models of social behavior might guide us to smile, maintain an appropriate distance, or avoid specific topics of conversation. We can categorize vast amounts of data, sort out the salient points, and then respond emotionally, cognitively, and behaviorally. Yet their downsides are too often clear. Implicit models are quickly accessed but prone to cognitive biases, logical errors, and incorrect assumptions. Implicit models can lead to discrimination because they are built from our personal experiences and cultural backgrounds, which are not universal and often more limited than we realize. Biases are usually unconscious and unexamined, which makes them difficult to identify and change. Implicit biases can affect our perceptions, decisions, and actions in a way that may be discriminatory, unfair, and, most of all, simply inaccurate (Payne & Cameron, 2013).

For example, someone might have an implicit model that "people who speak with a foreign accent are usually less intelligent." The person with this implicit model might unconsciously devalue the ideas of someone with an accent, even if there is no objective reason to do so. This kind of bias can lead to unfair treatment and discrimination and deprives both individuals of the potential richness of their interaction, talent, and collaboration.

Like many social behaviors, partisan political choices are often rooted in the implicit models that we hold, partly generated by our social identities (Clark & Winegard, 2020). Implicit models help us distill information rapidly based on our perceptions of who we are and what our friends are likely to believe. However, these models may also distort reality as we impose our beliefs on others. For instance, a person with an implicit model that their specific political party is morally correct will interpret information to support this belief. A person making this error shows evidence of a confirmation bias. On this cognitive bias, we tend to seek and favor information that confirms our pre-existing beliefs while ignoring or discounting data that challenges them. The opposite party's actions are seen as wrong and potentially evil. We can come to vilify anyone who disagrees with us, ascribing to them negative, almost inhuman characteristics, often because we think others who are similar to us are feeling that way too.

The "us-against-them" mentality, also known as the ingroup/outgroup dichotomy, is another aspect of our cognitive functioning rooted in our evolutionary past (Clark & Winegard, 2020). Anthropologists generally believe it was beneficial for our ancestors to work closely with their group and view outsiders with suspicion since outsiders could be threats. Today, this translates into political behavior through social categorization where we mentally categorize people into strict groups, often based on surface-level characteristics. For instance, if someone in the United States identifies as a Democrat, they may mentally categorize all Republicans as "them" and view them with suspicion or even hostility. The outgroup is often depicted as ethically inferior or evil as opposed to one's ingroup which is morally superior. Over time, these beliefs can become deeply ingrained, irrational, automatic, unconscious, and resistant to change.

Implicit models are often reflexively grounded in dichotomous thinking, a phenomenon that psychologists have long recognized. A standard implicit map that many people hold is the dichotomous view of Liberals vs. Conservatives. It is all "one side vs. another." People are on the Left or the Right with little, if any, overlap. In other words, they are either "Strongly similar" or "Vastly different" than me. These distortions can cause us to demonstrate bias in reasoning, which occurs when people are more willing to accept conclusions consistent with their sentiments (Calvillo & Harris, 2023).

A Spectrum Approach

> Once I realized that my clients' political views were as complex as my own, though perhaps in a different direction, I was able just to be more helpful. My own beliefs stayed out of the way.
>
> *(Mental Health Therapist, Columbus, Ohio)*

Politics, like many human endeavors, is infinitely complex and most people's views may not necessarily fit neatly into a simple binary of "left" vs. "right." There can be more variation and overlap than a strict binary view suggests. Viewing political sentiment as a spectrum of possible behaviors acknowledges this complexity. When we see political views as a dichotomy, it is easy to overgeneralize about people on the "other side." Viewing political orientation as a spectrum reminds us that there is a diversity of opinion within political groups. Not everyone fits the stereotype. Viewing political sentiment as a rigid dichotomy encourages "us vs. them" thinking.

A more flexible view of beliefs as a spectrum of possibilities emphasizes that people often have diverse perspectives, not necessarily divided into two opposing camps. Viewing behavior on a spectrum may build a degree of tolerance and understanding. A spectrum view allows for more compromise and incremental progress. People may share some beliefs with those on the "other side." A dichotomy promotes polarization and makes compromise harder, as political interaction in the United States and other countries has demonstrated in the last decade.

Most people can escape some of their tendencies toward dichotomized political thinking, at least temporarily. They can recognize that certain political beliefs may exist as "greater than" and "lesser than." Substantial data suggests that political ideas and ideologies fall on a normal bell curve, with most individuals clustering around the center (Jost, 2021). People who identify as strongly Left or Right likely represent the more extremes of this distribution. This is a view many of us endorse, at least sometimes, particularly in the United States and Britain, where there are few political parties. We often reference this model when we are not thinking dichotomously. It is undoubtedly better than the black-and-white "my side vs. others" that many people reflexively employ.

Recognition that political beliefs can exist on a spectrum or are generally more complex allows us to see that people can change their positions. They do not have to do so abruptly but can do so gradually and through time. There are, for example, predictable periods when people *as a group* become more conservative throughout life. These usually involve marriage and having children that typically occur in early adulthood. Social psychology literature contains many ways to make someone more liberal or conservative temporarily. For example, exposing someone to disgusting stimuli may make them temporarily—not permanently— more conservative. Exposing them to certain optimistic stimuli about the future may make them temporarily more progressive.

More permanent transformative experiences occasionally shift a person's position on the liberal-conservative spectrum. Yet, these are only sometimes predictable; they can be nonlinear and impossible to know in advance. For example, two individuals who fought in the same war and for the same side may have different political sentiments and agendas. One sees the need for a solid military and widespread patriotism. In contrast, the other sees the folly of armed conflict and the need to form a worldwide government to promote disarmament. Seemingly identical experiences may have opposite, nonlinear consequences.

While the normal distribution framework provides a helpful way to conceptualize political ideologies regarding their distribution within a population, it is crucial to recognize that political attitudes are sometimes more complex and dynamic than a simple linear spectrum. Many factors can influence people's beliefs, and political ideologies often evolve and adapt over time in response to individual experiences and changing societal, cultural, and economic circumstances. To make sense of this, consider some of the findings regarding the differences between people on the Left and the Right.

Science and Differences Between the Left and the Right

Most people think they know the "true" differences between liberals and conservatives. Again, this seems like common sense. Prominent areas of disagreement may include views on climate change, immigration, equality, nationalism, financial markets, security, religion, and social issues, such as gun control in the United States or Brexit, immigration, and the economy in Great Britain. However, our implicit models often lead us to assumptions about the personality, beliefs, or character of those with different opinions. We may make tremendous, unrecognized inferences based on a person's politics. These are often incorrect and prejudicial, keeping us from showing empathy or having a dialogue.

Individuals on both the Left and the Right are often quick to assign one another a variety of stereotypes. A pathway toward mitigating these implicit biases lies in our ability to discern the common beliefs underlying liberalism and conservatism. This endeavor can aid in dismantling the barriers that perpetuate the division between ingroups and outgroups, shedding light on the fundamental values that truly matter. Likewise, the tendency to label conservatives and progressives with stereotypical personality descriptions may be rectified by exploring scientific findings that reveal genuine distinctions in personality traits across the political spectrum. We can foster a more constructive dialogue that transcends these preconceived notions by embracing a more informed and nuanced perspective.

We may reduce political hostility and resentment by differentiating between implicit models and more explicit or evidence-based ones. Political partisans often describe a variety of abuses based on the alleged behaviors of those they feel are politically different. While research shows some general differences between people on the Left and Right regarding values and personality, there is a lot of diversity across the spectrum of beliefs (Haidt, 2012; Klein, 2020; Frisby, Redding, O'Donohue, & Lilienfeld, 2023). The key is to avoid assumptions and be open to different perspectives. Focusing on shared humanity and common goals helps bring people together.

There have been hundreds, quite literally, of different attitudes linked to the division between liberals and conservatives, and we are sure that there are probably many more. In many ways, attempting to chart attitudinal differences is similar to the early efforts of personality theorists who sought to find all the terms to describe individual differences. However, in the case of political views, many of these differences between the Left and the Right are somewhat inconsequential. Some are synonyms that tap the same constructs. Others have become very time bound. Others have "switched sides" through time, such as the role of the free market or a strong military.

Table 2.1 summarizes eight attitude clusters associated with people on the Left and Right that have received repeated empirical support and may be relevant for current clinical practice. These attitudes have been replicated in several studies and cultures. They are far from the only characteristics but may be the most common ones likely to matter to us in counseling or therapy.

People from conservative countries or more conservative U.S. citizens may tend to be pessimistic about the nature of humankind. The distrust of people on the Right for many social programs is rooted in the belief that they are not warranted or deserved and will be abused. Indeed, we can see this in Richard Nixon (a political conservative) during his presidency dismantling some of the Great Society programs enacted by Lyndon Johnson (a political liberal) in the United States in the 1970s.

Related to this, conservatives tend to distrust large government. An exception is in national defense, where they usually, though not always, wish to devote more resources. They typically favor less government because they feel governments tend to be corrupt and inefficient. They grow to favor reduced government regulation because they believe such laws are often ineffective and economically damaging. Usually, they think that government intervention weakens individual initiative and even personal morality. Contemporary conservatives tend to advocate strongly for the role of private enterprise and relatively unfettered capitalism.

Ironically, the modern conservative movement arose in the 19th century in response to populism and capitalism, wanting to restrict both. Regardless, conservatives usually favor tighter fiscal responsibility and generally lower taxes. Conservatives tend to see the market as efficient, and labor unions, regulations, and government as highly inefficient and ultimately harmful to society despite their seemingly good intentions.

Conservatives often believe that optimal personal freedom can only be guarded by vigilant individuals protecting themselves, their families, and their communities. People cannot and should not expect the government to defend them, except for matters of national defense. Liberals are also concerned about losing freedom but often apply these concerns more generally to underrepresented groups or populations. They tend to rely on the national government and local institutions for protection from threats.

Conservatives often believe classic morality, including that from traditional scriptures, is best for society and should be upheld by social institutions. Behaviors that they support may include prohibiting or restricting LGBTQ+ marriages, reducing or prohibiting abortion, banning recreational drug use (but only in some American segments), or (in some cases) limiting the roles and

TABLE 2.1 Attitudes associated with conservatives and liberals

Attitude	Conservatives/more right leaning people	Liberals/more left-leaning people
Feelings about Human Nature	Often less trusting	Often more positive and trusting
Sentiment about Government	Distrustful, favors small and local government	Generally, support a more active government capable of enacting widespread change
Economy	Often favor free-market capitalism, advocating for lower taxes to stimulate economic growth	Government oversight and regulations are needed to ensure fairness
Individual liberties	Individual liberties within the bounds of Judeo-Christian values are the hallmark of a democracy	Government is necessary to protect the liberties of disenfranchised groups, such as racial, ethnic, and sexual minorities
Morality	Typically favors traditional morality, such as in Abrahamic scriptures or the Quran (in Islamic countries), which eschews abortion, same-sex marriage, and transgender rights	Typically leans toward individual freedom in moral and social decisions
Self-interest and responsibility vs. other interest	Self-interest is positive and maximizes social good	Group effort and unselfishness maximize social good
Hierarchies	Some people are more worthy or valuable than others, hence, hierarchies are natural and necessary	All people are philosophically equal and should be treated that way; hierarchies should be avoided as much as possible
Social cohesion	Society has static demands. Often, nostalgia for the past. Society exists primarily to enforce morality and limit human excesses	Society is dynamic. The future can be better than the past. Society exists to maximize human potential

rights of women and minorities in society. Furthermore, conservatives may tend to believe that humans are primarily self-motivated and self-interested. Economic progress does not usually come from cooperation but most typically from individuals acting in self-interest. Likewise, the conservative tradition is rooted in the belief that some people are naturally superior to others and that hierarchies are necessary and positive. It may openly argue for the superiority of some groups. A liberal tradition generally eschews these lines of thinking and is instead focused on eradicating inequality and providing opportunities for oppressed or marginalized populations. They view cooperation and coalition building, such as local activism, as a means to influence political change.

Issues and concerns that define the liberal-conservative divisions may change through time. Conservatism in the United States became prominent with their platform against populism and laissez-faire capitalism. Ironically, today, many conservatives are populists, and the support for unrestricted capitalism is generally most robust among the Right.

Liberalism arose as a system that is based on respecting everyone's rights. More recently, liberals are more likely to be at the forefront of "cancel culture," ostracizing and attempting to silence people who do not have similar values. While this is often difficult for people on the Left to see, it is undeniable. Ironically, political inclinations designed to protect everyone frequently stifle some viewpoints. More progressive liberals sometimes become arbiters of censorship of those who have more traditional or conservative perspectives. We see this on some college campuses where right-leaning speakers or faculty are the target of protests.

Since the 1950s, the Right has been the party of strong defense and military interventionism in the United States. More recently, there is often an about-face, with people on the Right returning to the isolationism of the early 20th century. Historically, the left wing has advocated for more government intervention in the economy, including social welfare programs, wealth redistribution, and regulations to protect workers and consumers. In recent years, however, some right-wing movements have adopted protectionist economic policies and emphasized the interests of workers over corporations. These sentiments were traditionally associated with the Left. Defining critical issues between the Left and Right can be difficult because they often change. For example, some on the Left recently began advocating for a return to the gold standard to back currency in the United States. This demand was previously strongly associated with the pundits on the Right. Concern about government fluoridation of public drinking water, once seen as an example of extreme Right-wing conspiracy thinking from the 1960s, has now resurfaced on the Left. Those opposing use of vaccines all over the world are both liberal and conservative, much to the dismay of more empirically minded medical authorities.

Psychological Differences Between Liberals and Conservatives

> If I could understand liberals, and where they are coming from, I genuinely think I could treat them better. But their beliefs just don't make any sense to me.
>
> *(Compulsive Gambling Counselor, Oregon)*

> If I could really get inside the head of a conservative ... I mean, why are their personalities the way they are? If I could answer this I could probably treat them with more success. But they're a mystery to me.
>
> *(Addiction Counselor, Arizona)*

One way to make sense of the differences between the Left and the Right is to look for psychological traits that co-occur with patterns of political beliefs. Personalities and psychological traits of liberals and conservatives have been the subject of extensive research in psychology and neuroscience since at least the 1940s. Over 300 traits have been highlighted in the literature, substantially beyond our current discussion. More seem to be found every month and often make the popular press or wind up as crude internet memes. Almost all these traits have only a small or, at best, a moderate correlation with indicators of political affiliation. They are also, at best, tendencies or probabilities that do not account for much of the total observed variance in personality. Regardless, the following differences are probably the most important for counseling and psychotherapy. Table 2.2 highlights some common *potential* psychological differences between liberals and conservatives supported by multiple studies. Again, the statistical effect sizes for these are typically small-to-moderate.

A summary of research has shown that people who score higher in openness to experience, a personality trait that includes preferring novelty, diversity, and intellectual curiosity, tend to have more liberal political beliefs. In contrast, conservatives tend to score lower on this trait. Instead, conservatives often score higher on conscientiousness, which involves a preference for order, structure, and stability (De Neve, 2015). This might be linked to a conservative inclination for traditionalism, established social norms, and authority over ambiguity. Liberals are often considered more tolerant of risk and uncertainty, while conservatives are more risk averse. This can affect attitudes toward social change and policy. These correlations are in the small to moderate range.

There is some evidence that people on the Left are somewhat less fearful, although these findings are complex. It may be that conservatives have more specific fears about certain areas. It was thought conservatives feared contamination, but their response to viruses, notably COVID-19 and other viruses, does not support this theory. It does not appear that either side tends toward excessive generalized anxiety or other psychiatric illnesses. Neither side

TABLE 2.2 Psychological differences between liberals and conservatives

Trait	Liberals	Conservatives
Openness	Often more novelty-seeking and open to change and creative pursuits	Usually less novelty-seeking and comfortable with traditions
Tolerance of risk	Often more open to risk	Characteristically, less tolerant of personal and social risks
Conscientiousness	Frequently less conscientious	Frequently more conscientious
Perceived threats	Less sensitive to threats involving group solidarity and security	Often more threat-sensitive toward self and groups
Disgust sensitivity	Frequently lower	Frequently higher
Authoritarianism/hierarchies	Typically, less tolerant of authorities with many exceptions such as medical professionals	Often defer to hierarchy as the natural order
Traits associated with traditional Male/Female roles	More androgynous	Usually more gender stereotyped

tends to lack boldness. Neurological studies discussed below have found that conservatives may be more sensitive to disgust. Again, these correlations tend to be small.

Reasons why conservatives prefer and defer to hierarchy and may be more authoritarian on their extremes are still not well known despite almost 100 years of study (Duckitt, 2019). This finding has been replicated repeatedly. The correlation could be due to findings that conservatives may be more sensitive to some aspects of fear. However, more current data suggests against this, at least in American samples (Clifton & Kerry, 2023). Other recent research emphasizes that people who identify as politically liberal tend to be more empathetic and more androgynous in their interests (Hassan et al., 2018). Conservatives may grow to be more gender stereotyped, perhaps over time or perhaps through the process of experiencing socialization from more traditional backgrounds. Therefore, they may develop into people who are more comfortable with those who assume traditional gender roles. Again, the emphasis on tradition and comfort with the familiar should be viewed as an emerging theme.

Both liberals and conservatives often provide evidence that their side has a higher intelligence quotient or other highly desirable cognitive abilities that set them apart. However, this type of research is mired in so many confounding variables that it is not helpful for science, much less for the clinician. It may, however, make an appealing meme for social media, which might be the primary intention.

There is increasing, though still emerging, evidence that *some* differences between the Left and the Right are based partly on genetic factors. This complex and controversial area has been reviewed by Hibbing, Smith, and Alford (2014) and, more recently, by Jost (2021). It is obvious that there is no single "politics gene." Traits that are normally distributed in a population have a multigenetic basis. Unlike those controlled by a single autosomal gene, multigenetic characteristics are influenced by the interaction of numerous genetic factors, which tend to produce a bell-shaped, normal distribution in the population when aggregated. Environmental factors often interact with multiple genetic factors, further contributing to the continuous variation observed in these traits, as opposed to the distinct phenotypes typically associated with single gene (autosomal) traits. Like so many other human characteristics, it's a dance between nature and nurture.

Epigenetic factors are also important although we are clearly only beginning to understand this complex process. Epigenetics refers to molecular processes that regulate how genes are expressed without altering the DNA sequence. Experiences and environmental exposures can lead to epigenetic changes that influence behavior and psychology. Epigenetics involves chemical changes to DNA or associated proteins that determine whether genes are turned on or off, thereby regulating their expression.

We are far from understanding both the genetics and epigenetics of political affiliation. There is still too little here to guide the therapist who works with people who experience political polarization. Regardless of genetics or epigenetic influences, therapy may succeed in teaching someone how to be kinder and more respectful in how they communicate with dissimilar others. It can help reduce the malignant pettiness that has increasingly characterized all parts of the political spectrum. Therapy and counseling will not likely turn liberals into conservatives or Right-wingers toward the Left. It can, however, make people of any political orientation kinder, more reflective, more able to listen, and more tolerant.

There are many other differences between people on the Left and the Right. There is also some evidence that there may be differences in balances between specific neurotransmitters that differentiate the Left from the Right. Lieberman and Long (2018) hypothesize that liberals are more dopamine-driven while conservatives are more noradrenergically based. Dopamine is often associated with pleasure, but these authors note that it is also related to desire, seeking out what we want, and not being content with what we have. Norepinephrine (noradrenaline) is a neurotransmitter in the body's stress response. It helps to increase alertness, focus attention, and prepare the body for "fight or flight." Elevated aspects of noradrenergic response might explain why conservatives are more prone to anxiety about ingroup fears. They may also have more neurotransmitters associated with anxiousness about the future. On the other hand, they are more likely to be happy with the status quo and perhaps happier in general. Again, these are tendencies that combine with environmental factors and are somewhat speculative.

We contend that regardless of social learning, early experiences, psychodynamics, and genetic causes of political orientation, members of humanity must treat each other with decency and respect. This should not be in the least controversial. However, if we accept this belief, then the causes of the liberal/conservative divide matter much less and are basically of less importance than our common humanity and shared experiences.

Beyond the Left/Right Axis

This simple distinction of a single dimension of political orientation works reasonably well in many situations. It is most people's "go-to" model, including most mental health providers. However, it does not answer more complex questions. For example, one commonly debated on the Internet is: "Were the Nazis Leftwing or Rightwing?" Both people on the Left and Right are quick to shoulder Nazi politics and morality to the other side. Perhaps more challenging, still, is how political Libertarians fit our model. How about people who have a variety of conflicting views? For example, in the United Kingdom, consider a Scottish person who favored Brexit and supported immigrant controls, is a proponent of social welfare programs, and strongly supports Scotland's independence. Where do they stand on our spectrum of Left vs. Right? As with many dichotomies in human behavior, there are many people who don't clearly fit on either side of the spectrum.

A dimensional framework for political attitudes can often provide a more nuanced understanding of the complexities of political ideology. This framework can be helpful for the counselor or therapist because it allows even more flexibility. Such a framework recognizes that political beliefs often cannot be fully captured along a single left-right spectrum and instead considers two or more dimensions that shape individuals' political attitudes. It allows us additional ways of avoiding stereotyping and understanding the complexities of peoples' characteristic ways of responding to political questions.

The Political Compass model is an improvement over a flat line continuum. It plots political attitudes along two axes: economic left wing-right wing) and social (authoritarian-libertarian). The economic axis represents attitudes toward monetary policy, ranging from Left (more state intervention and economic equality) to Right (free-market principles and limited government intervention). The social axis captures attitudes toward personal freedoms and social issues, ranging from authoritarian (emphasis on traditional values and social order) to libertarian (emphasis on individual rights and personal liberties). This framework allows for a more comprehensive understanding of political attitudes by acknowledging that people can hold a mix of economic and social beliefs. For example, someone may hold left-leaning views about the need for subsidized housing but simultaneously have very socially conservative values about sexual behavior or banning violent video games.

Other core dimensions have been suggested to underlie the liberal–conservative continuum. These include attitudes toward inequality on one axis and social change vs. tradition on another (Jost, Glaser, Kruglanski, & Sulloway, 2003). These researchers also stress that these dimensions are socially learned attitudes and can be modified by environmental factors, such as family, peer groups, or social norms. Jost et al. (2021) believe that political attitudes are social cognitions, meaning that they have been discovered in a social context through modeling and, as such, can be changed to some extent.

In the middle of the last century, the prolific and controversial personality researcher Hans Eysenck proposed a different two-axis model. Eysenck (1954) included a dimension of "Tough vs. Tendermindedness." Tough-minded individuals are rational, pragmatic, and interested in objective facts and evidence. In contrast, tender-minded individuals are more emotional and empathetic and value subjective experiences and feelings. A second dimension is "radicalism" vs. "conservatism." Radical individuals are described as open to change, interested in new ideas, and more likely to challenge authority and established norms. In contrast, conservative individuals are more inclined to maintain the status quo, respect tradition and power, and be cautious about change.

According to Eysenck, these two dimensions are relatively independent, meaning that someone can be any combination of them. Using these two dimensions, Eysenck could describe different political belief systems and ideologies. For example, he suggested that tough-minded and conservative people tend to be more right-wing. In contrast, those who are both tender-minded and radical tend to be left-wing-oriented. Tender-minded and conservative are who we might now call libertarians. Tough-minded and liberal-produce communists or radicals.

Our current variation of these two-dimensional models that we have found clinically useful avoids the labels of "Left and Right" and "Liberal and Conservative" and instead focuses on two factors. One is Trust vs. Distrust, which we believe sums up belief in authority. The second is the Preservation of the Past vs. Optimism for the Future. This model is still heuristic but avoids categorizing clients who wish to escape what they may perceive as stereotyping or being labeled a liberal or conservative.

Multifactor Model of Moral Values

Sometimes, our maps may become too rigid and impede understanding of our clients' thoughts or feelings. Traditional "right vs. left" distinctions may be either too restrictive or simply irrelevant. Two dimensional models may fail to address clients' underlying moral values and how that affects their way of interacting with the world. Many other models of political division may be more helpful to clinicians and counselors. Milton Rokeach's (1961, 1973) highly influential theory of liberals and conservatives can be understood based on his broader work in the field of values and belief systems. Rokeach posited that liberals and conservatives differ fundamentally in the core values and beliefs that shape their attitudes and behaviors. For instance, conservatives might prioritize values such as tradition, stability, and security, emphasizing respect for authority and social hierarchy. In contrast, liberals might highly value progress, equality, and social change, advocating for social justice and individual rights. This theoretical framework underscores the psychological underpinnings of political ideologies, explaining how deep-seated beliefs and values contribute to the distinct worldviews of liberals and conservatives.

Kerlinger (1972), a well-known multivariate theorist, also proposed that instead of a continuum, liberals and conservatives are tuned to different sets of values. Kerlinger's theory on liberal/conservative differences focused on "criterial referents." According to his theory, liberals and conservatives tend to have different criteria or referents, which are the fundamental beliefs, values, or issues central to their ideological identity. For conservatives, these referents might include religion, economic conservatism, traditionalism, and morality. In contrast, liberals may have different referents. Their referents might include social justice, individual rights, and progressive ideas about social issues. The core idea is that these criteria referents shape and differentiate the social attitudes and ideological perspectives of liberals and conservatives, implying that their worldviews are structured around different fundamental principles and concerns.

The renown social psychologist Jonathan Haidt has reflected these ideas in one of the more influential theories in political psychology of the last 20 years. He presents an empirically derived model that may also be clinically useful. Haidt's theory, like Kerlinger's, is based on the idea that different moral values and emotions shape diverse political beliefs (Haidt, 2012). Haidt proposes that people use six universal moral values to evaluate their actions and the actions of others: care/harm, fairness/cheating, loyalty/betrayal, authority/subversion, sanctity/degradation, and liberty/oppression. According to Haidt's research, liberals and conservatives emphasize these moral values differently, which explains why they often hold different political beliefs.

Haidt argues that liberals prioritize the importance of care/harm and fairness/cheating above other moral concerns. In contrast, conservatives prioritize all six areas: care, fairness, loyalty, authority, sanctity, and liberty. Haidt also suggests that liberals and conservatives have different emotional and psychological tendencies that shape their political beliefs. He indicates that liberals tend to be more open to new experiences, more likely to question authority, and more concerned with social justice and equality issues. Conservatives tend to be more focused on preserving traditional social structures, are more sensitive to threats to social order, and are more concerned with group identity and loyalty issues.

Based on Haidt's theory, changing the priorities people assign to these moral values may be possible. However, we do not know whether this will likely result in a sustainable change. We also question whether it is ethical if the client does not wish for their values to change or whether changes occur without awareness. A reminder here that the focus of therapy is not to change a client's political positions, rather to understand how they impact the person's life for better or worse.

Facts Don't Matter: A Partisan Identity Model

One of the more clinically valuable models may help explain how people, regardless of their pre-existing personalities or left-right orientation, become dominated by political motivation. Mason (2018) argues that there is a distinction between firmly held political beliefs and the process of developing a partisan identity. A spectrum or a continuum can best represent political beliefs. Partisan identity is something more. It occurs through a progressive process of sorting and self-definition that happens over time. Partisan identities are based on group affiliations, approval, and what we think people like us should believe. It occurs through a process of "partisan sorting." Partisan sorting occurs when people separate themselves, first into parties that match their ideology and then into progressively more isolative, like-minded groups that exclude people we even suspect might hold different views than us. This becomes an upward spiral of self-selected sameness and exclusiveness characterized by suspicion and hostility to anyone who deviates from our way of thinking. Most recently, the exaggerated and strident political differences that have dominated our divisions are not so much about disagreements regarding fundamental political beliefs, but arise because partisan identities have been socially constructed through increased sorting and affiliation with those we think we should emulate.

Ultimately, this gives rise to the well-known concept of *identity politics*. Identity politics refers to organizing and mobilizing around the interests and perspectives of particular social or cultural groups, often based on characteristics such as race, ethnicity, gender, sexual orientation, religion, or other aspects of personal identity. It involves asserting group-specific struggles, experiences, and demands within the broader political and social landscape. Identity politics is associated with *psychological tribalism*, embraced by both the Left and the Right. Tribalism in politics and government refers to political groups that become more focused on allegiance to their own "tribe" (political party, faction, etc.) rather than focusing on compromise or the overall good of society. Some key signs and impacts of tribalism in government include hyper-partisanship, where one party reflexively opposes the other party's positions and goals, even if they may overlap. There is an "us vs. them" mentality, discussed in Chapter 1, which as much as we try to avoid seems instinctive. Sadly, it will be a recurrent theme throughout much of this volume.

The results of partisan process and tribalism are often damaging to rational governing. Politicians may increasingly become more motivated to beat the other party than to pass effective legislation. Scoring political points can override sound policymaking. Hurting the other side is more important than meaningful compromise to address important problems. There is little effort to find common ground or compromise. Debates become polarized and gridlocked. Supporters are loyal to their party above principles or consistency. Critics of the party are attacked, even if they have valid concerns. Compromise is seen as surrender rather than a way to assure that legislation or policy is more balanced.

As both the Left and the Right point out about the other side, politicians may engage in tribal signaling through rhetoric, symbols, and social media posts to show allegiance to the party "tribe." Group affiliation is prized over individual nuance. Facts, data, and policy specifics can become less relevant than supporting the tribe's narrative. Loyalty to the tribe's beliefs is valued over objective truth, the needs of the country, and the welfare of its people.

The rise of social media and online platforms has facilitated the formation of hyperpolarized communities based on shared identities and experiences. These platforms allow individuals to connect, organize, and raise awareness about issues affecting their specific communities and causes. Online activism has played a significant role in promoting identity politics and fostering collective mobilization.

Decreasing tribalism and partisan identity may well be a possible goal for clients and perhaps ourselves as well. Attempting to influence change in a person's underlying political orientation through therapy is certainly an ethical violation unless that is a goal explicitly stated by the client. The degree, however, to which they express this orientation as a function of social influence may be amenable to change. It may be possible for people to dialogue in therapy with others who are different and discover views both the therapist and client previously failed to consider. While the first goal of this book is to encourage therapists and counselors to gain understanding of the way that politics is affecting the therapy space, the second goal is to convince them that they can serve as *dialogue agents*. In other chapters, we will discuss how a Partisan Identity arises and discuss steps that we can take to encourage dialogue and reduce tribal hostilities.

Finally, some scholars have argued that the concepts of Left and Right are essentially arbitrary. Labels switch through time and are flexible. While we do not fully endorse this idea, there may be much truth to it, and yesterday's conservatives may be tomorrow's progressives.

Summary

Chapter 2 explores the psychological and ideological differences between liberals and conservatives, emphasizing the complexity of political identities beyond a simple left-right dichotomy. The chapter explored the impact of implicit models and stereotypes on understanding political orientations, highlighting how these perceptions influence interactions and counseling practices. We delve into various models and theories that attempt to categorize political beliefs, showing how these frameworks can help psychotherapy by fostering empathy and understanding across political divides.

We also examined the role of psychological traits, moral values, and genetic factors in shaping political ideologies, suggesting that many factors, including personality traits and socialization processes, influence political beliefs. Although our review is not comprehensive, we attempt to challenge the notion of a binary political spectrum, proposing instead a multifaceted approach to understanding political attitudes that accommodates a broader range of viewpoints and complexities. This nuanced perspective encourages the recognition of shared humanity and common goals, aiming to mitigate polarization and enhance dialogue across ideological lines.

References

Calvillo, D. P., & Harris, J. D. (2023). Exposure to headlines as questions reduces illusory truth for subsequent headlines. *Journal of Applied Research in Memory and Cognition*, *12*(3), 335–343. https://doi.org/10.1037/mac0000056

Cattell, R. B., & Kline, P. (1977). *The scientific analysis of personality and motivation.* New York: Academic Press.

Chamberlain, L. (2021). *Practicing psychotherapy: Lessons on helping patients and growing as a professional.* New York: Routledge.

Clark, C. J., & Winegard, B. M. (2020). Tribalism in war and peace: The nature and evolution of ideological epistemology and its significance for modern social science. *Psychological Inquiry*, *31*(1), 1–22. https://doi.org/10.1080/1047840X.2020.1721233

Clifton, J. D., & Kerry, N. (2023). Belief in a dangerous world does not explain substantial variance in political attitudes, but other world beliefs do. Social Psychological and Personality Science, 13(5). https://doi.org/10.1177/19485506221119

De Neve, J. E. (2015). Personality, childhood experience, and political ideology. *Political Psychology*, *36*(1), 55–73. https://doi.org/10.1111/pops.12075

Duckitt, J. (2019). *The social psychology of prejudice.* Oxford: Praeger.

Eysenck, H. J. (1954). The science of personality: Nomothetic. *Psychological Review*, *61*(5), 339–342. https://doi.org/10.1037/h0058333

Frisby, C. L., Redding, R. E., O'Donohue, W. T., & Lilienfeld, S.O. (Eds.) (2023). *Ideological and political bias in psychology: Nature, scope and solutions.* Cham, Switzerland: Springer.

Haidt, J. (2012). *The righteous mind: Why good people are divided by politics and religion.* New York: Vintage.

Hassan, G., Brouillette-Alarie, S., Seraphin, A., et.al. (2018). Exposure to extremist online content could lead to violent radicalization: A systematic review of empirical evidence. International Journal of Development. https://doi.org/10.3233/DEV-170233

Hibbing, J. R., Smith, K. B., & Alford, J. R. (2014). *Predisposed: Liberals, conservatives, and the biology of political differences.* New York, NY: Routledge.

Jost, J. T. (2021). *Left and right: The psychological significance of a political distinction.* Oxford University Press.

Jost, J. T., Glaser, J., Kruglanski, A. W., & Sulloway, F. J. (2003). Political conservatism and motivated social cognition. *Psychological Bulletin, 129*(3). https://doi.org/10.1037/0033-2909.129.3.339

Kerlinger, F. N. (1972). The structure and content of social attitude referents: A preliminary study. *Educational and Psychological Measurement, 32,* 613–618.

Klein, E. (2020). *Why we're polarized.* New York: Avid Reader Press.

Lieberman, D. Z., & Long, M. E. (2018). *The molecule of more: How a single chemical in your brain drives love, sex, and creativity—And will determine the fate of the human race.* BenBella Books.

Mason, L. (2018). *Uncivil agreement: How politics became our identity.* Chicago: University of Chicago Press.

3

POLITICAL TO PARTISAN

How We Got Here

Not New: A Synopsis of the Current Split

Political divisiveness is not unique to the United States. It is a phenomenon increasingly observed in various democracies worldwide. It is not, by any means, a modern occurrence. In his book "Why We're Polarized" (2020), Ezra Klein provides a history of America's descent into division and dysfunction. Political divides similar to our own and have been well documented since ancient Greece and arguably before. For example, in ancient Greece, Sparta was generally conservative, while Athens and other city-states were more politically progressive. By the time of the Roman Empire, the notion of the comparatively progressive populists and the conservative traditionalists, for example, Cato, were well established.

Today, however, democracies, both new and old, are confronting internal and external challenges that contribute to increasing polarization. With its Brexit referendum, the United Kingdom experienced significant political divisions, paralleling the political polarity in the United States. The Brexit vote revealed deep divisions within British society regarding political alignment and cultural, regional, and generational aspects. Other European countries, like Spain with its Catalonia independence movement and France with the Yellow Vest protests, have also faced political divisiveness on various issues. The political situation in Germany may be difficult for an outsider to understand but seems dominated by more extreme Left and Right factions.

In Asia, India has seen increased political polarization, particularly around issues of religious and cultural identity. Similarly, Brazil and Argentina experienced heightened political divisiveness, especially during recent

DOI: 10.4324/9781032651217-3

presidential elections. These examples illustrate that political polarization is a global phenomenon affecting democracies worldwide, often driven by a combination of social, economic, and cultural factors.

Because the authors are from the United States, where the divide seems to be the most salient, we will primarily focus on the development of the American divide, with a brief discussion of the United Kingdom and Canada. However, we believe that increasing partisan politicization applies to various democracies and will likely increase throughout the world, adding to difficulties in counseling and psychotherapy practices in various countries and contexts.

History of the Divide in America

The evolution of the current political divide between the left and the right in the United States did not occur overnight. As indicated, some of its roots are as deep as ancient history. However, from the 1980s through the 2020s, the division seems to have accelerated, jumpstarted by various social, economic, technological, and political factors. Historians, political scientists, psychologists, sociologists, and other behavioral and social scientists disagree on the exact causes. There is, however, a consensus that several events helped shape this current situation.

The 1960s and 1970s were a period of rapid social and cultural change in America, characterized by several movements pushing the country toward a more progressive and liberal direction. This era saw greater activism around civil rights, women's equality, sexual freedom, and anti-war protests. The civil rights movement, seeking to end segregation and achieve full equality for African Americans, peaked with landmarks like the March on Washington, the passage of the Civil Rights Act of 1964, and the Voting Rights Act of 1965. The Women's Liberation Movement expanded opportunities for women in society and the workplace through feminist activism, the advent of the birth control pill, and the legalization of abortion in 1973. The sexual revolution brought more permissive attitudes toward sex, birth control, pornography, and LGBTQ+ rights as the counterculture rejected strict sexual mores. Gay rights, simmering for so long, fully emerged following the Stonewall Riots in 1969 and subsequent events. One outcome of this social movement was the American Psychiatric Association's decision in 1973 to remove "Homosexuality" as a mental disorder from the Diagnostic and Statistical Manual II, 2nd edition. (American Psychiatric Association, 1973).

Meanwhile, anti-war protests coalesced around opposition to the Vietnam War, with youth activists aligned against the military draft. Expanded civil liberties like free speech were strengthened through court cases. The progressive grassroots mobilization of the 1960s and 1970s challenged traditional hierarchies. It nudged the country toward more significant social and cultural liberalism.

In the United States, this period also represented increasing political liberalization by both major political parties. This was true even for Republican President Richard Nixon, a previously staunch Conservative who implemented several progressive policies during his tenure. He established the Environmental Protection Agency (EPA) and signed landmark environmental legislation, such as the Clean Air Act, marking significant advancements in ecological protection. Nixon also enforced desegregation in Southern schools, supported the Equal Rights Amendment for women (still not passed in the United States), and proposed health insurance reform and a form of guaranteed minimum income. These policies reflected an approach to social issues that transcended traditional conservative ideology.

There has been a substantial shift since Nixon's reach toward the center. Both parties have shifted away from the political center in the United States between 1980 and 2025. There is presently almost no overlap between the two parties, which is rare by the historical standards of this or many other nations. Even when bi-partisan legislation manages to be created, such as the 2024 effort by both parties working together to propose a balanced immigration policy, political pressures to avoid compromise assured that it would not be enacted.

The Cultural Divide in Britain

Great Britain was drifting leftward after World War II, at least until the election of Margaret Thatcher. In the immediate post-war period, the Labour Party under Clement Attlee came to power, focusing on building a comprehensive welfare state and implementing industrial reforms. This era saw significant nationalization of key industries and the establishment of the National Health Service, reflecting a solid progressive shift in economic and social policies, emphasizing state intervention and social welfare. This trend continued with the post-war consensus, a period of shared agreement between the major political parties on the importance of a mixed economy, nationalization, and a robust welfare state. This consensus, which lasted until the late 1970s, signified a general leftward inclination in British politics. The arrival of Margaret Thatcher in 1979 marked a significant shift as her government initiated a series of right-leaning reforms, including privatization of state industries and a move away from the principles of the post-war consensus.

The 1980s marked a significant era for the conservative movement in Great Britain. In the United States, President Ronald Reagan's administration heralded this change through "Reaganomics," a set of policies that emphasized tax cuts, deregulation, increased military spending, and reduced government spending on social programs. Prime Minister Margaret Thatcher's government may have predated this conservative wave in Great Britain. Thatcherism, as it was known, focused on free-market policies, the privatization of state-owned industries, and a reduction in the power of trade unions. This approach aimed to tackle the economic issues plaguing Britain, such as high inflation and unemployment. The Thatcher era arguably revitalized the British economy, marked by increased productivity and economic growth. However, it also led to increased inequality and social unrest, with many people noting that there was a disinvestment in human capital. Nonetheless, these economic policies firmly established the conservative ideology in British politics, influencing successive governments. In the summer of 2024, Britian saw the rise again of a more liberal coalition and the more liberal-leaning Labour Party succeeded in reclaiming political control of the country.

On the international front, the conservative movement of the 1980s significantly impacted global politics and military strategies. Great Britain had a success with the Falkland War, which was seen internationally as vindication of the conservative policies of Mrs. Thatcher. At the same time, the United States, under Reagan, took a hardline stance against the Soviet Union, dubbing it the "Evil Empire" and significantly increasing military spending. This approach, combined with strategic economic policies, contributed to the weakening of the Soviet economy and its eventual collapse, marking the end of the Cold War. The downfall of the Soviet Union in the early 1990s was seen as confirmation that these policies were correct as intellectual heirs of Mr. Reagan and Mrs. Thatcher remind us.

The 1990s Onward: America, Britain, and Canada

The 1990s marked a significant shift, particularly in American politics, highlighted by an increasingly polarized electorate. While some of this was in response to Regan, other vital factors emerged independently. One was the rise of "Single-Issue Politics," where political interest groups were driven by one overriding theme. The increase of single-issue groups, often with extreme views, began to push parties away from the center. In the United States, issues like abortion, gun rights, and environmental policies became litmus tests for political allegiance, superseding broader policy platforms and, subsequently, the ability to compromise.

The 1990s United States also witnessed a closer alignment between conservative politics and evangelical Christianity, notably with the Moral Majority and Christian Coalition, leading to more ideologically driven policies. While the extreme right has long had a connection with religion, this connection has become more prominent and more confined to a specific type of belief. At one time, highly conservative views were endorsed by the Catholic Church and by extreme protestant factions. However, by the 1990s, the Evangelical and conservative Christian communities supporting right-wing causes had become much more embedded and progressively intolerant of diverse opinions.

The emergence of cable news networks in the United States, like Fox News and MSNBC, which often presented news with a particular political slant, began to create echo chambers, reinforcing viewers' pre-existing beliefs. Perhaps even more forceful was the reverberation from talk radio in the United States, particularly popular on the Right. The internet's infancy in the 1990s altered how information was consumed and shared. It also became a means for anyone to share their political and social beliefs, theories, and biases. Its full political impact, however, would not be realized until later decades.

The decline in the American manufacturing sector, accelerated by progressive policies, added to the division. Many people saw themselves as hopeless and helpless, sold out by politicians whose interests were in catering to an elite group that many citizens could not join. Factory jobs, which supported millions of households from the Industrial Revolution onward, were either becoming more automated or being moved overseas where labor costs were lower. The middle class, which was created in large part by factory workers, began to struggle.

The 2000s intensified the political divide, influenced by 9/11 and its aftermath. The response to the 9/11 attacks and subsequent wars in Afghanistan and Iraq created deep divisions in American public opinion, with debates over security, freedom, and America's role in the world. A sense of vulnerability and fear promoted increased spending on national security and the military. Local police forces became similar to military operations.

The proliferation of the internet and the rise of social media platforms like Facebook and Twitter significantly impacted political discourse, allowing for the rapid spread of information and misinformation. In both the United States and Great Britain, issues around race and heated debates over immigration policy further polarized opinions. The financial crisis and the subsequent Great Recession exacerbated economic inequalities in many countries. They heightened resentment toward perceived government mismanagement and corporate greed. This increased cynicism and decreased tolerance for believing the government was a force for human good. It also resulted in substantial psychological dysfunction in people who experienced disastrous economic conditions. In the United States, economic recovery from the 2008 downturn was uneven, leading to increased frustration among working-class individuals who felt left behind by globalization and technological change. In Great Britain, economic recovery was even slower, further adding to political discontent.

The 2010s saw the culmination of these trends lead to heightened political antagonism and distrust. This era saw a significant decline in critical thinking, with emotional appeals and confirmation biases dominating the debate. Political discourse became increasingly vitriolic, with personal attacks and harsh rhetoric becoming more commonplace and socially tolerated. By the 2010s, the internet and social media had become central to political campaigning and discourse, with platforms often serving as echo chambers and breeding grounds for extremist views. Magazines and newspapers stopped publication, victims of the internet as a source for news, and some venture capitalistic practices. This resulted in fewer news sources and those that survived tended to have a more partisan viewpoint, advocating political dogma.

In the United Kingdom, Brexit became a dominant theme that many people in the United States still cannot comprehend. The Brexit referendum passed by a narrow margin of 51.9% to 48.1%, exposing significant divisions within the United Kingdom. Proponents of Brexit argued it would allow the United Kingdom to take back control of its sovereignty from EU institutions and restrict immigration. However, opponents contended Brexit would have disastrous economic consequences and isolate the United Kingdom diplomatically. The close referendum result showed Britain starkly divided on whether to remain in or leave the EU, and this division continues.

In the United States, racial tensions continued to be a divisive issue, with the rise of movements like Black Lives Matter in response to police brutality and systemic racism. Simultaneously, anti-immigrant sentiment and xenophobia were stoked by certain political factions in many countries in Europe and Asia. Issues around immigration policies are contentious in many countries and people remain divided about how to address these concerns.

Evidence of foreign interference in elections, particularly the 2016 U.S. presidential election, raised concerns about the vulnerability of democratic processes to external manipulation. These concerns remain unresolved many years later, with charges and countercharges still standing. Regardless, it is clear that powerful special interests used social media to spread divisive rumors and disinformation in ways that were not imaginable a few years previously. There was also a growing perception among many voters on both the Right and the Left in many countries that political elites were out of touch with the ordinary person's needs and concerns, leading to increased distrust in traditional political institutions.

The COVID-19 pandemic, beyond its global health implications, significantly deepened political polarization, particularly in the United States, where responses to the pandemic often aligned with political ideologies. Similar trends were observed in the United Kingdom and elsewhere, though not as pronounced as in the United States. Liberals and conservatives differed markedly in their perceptions of the pandemic's risks, levels of trust in politicians and government measures, and adherence to health guidelines. A study in early 2020 showed that liberals perceived a higher risk from COVID-19 compared to conservatives and placed less trust in politicians and health experts to manage the crisis effectively (Smith, 2022). This divergence in perception and response can be attributed to varying media consumption habits and ideological beliefs, where conservatives tended to downplay the severity of the pandemic or viewed restrictive measures as infringements on personal freedoms. The pandemic thus became a flashpoint, exacerbating existing political divides and fostering an environment where public health measures were interpreted through a partisan lens.

This political polarization was not just limited to perceptions but extended to the very nature of the response to the pandemic. In the United States, partisan divides led to differing approaches to lockdowns, mask mandates, and vaccination campaigns in states that were more liberal or conservative. Such division was reflected in the public's behavior and attitudes toward these measures. For instance, the vaccine rollout became entangled in political identity, with conservatives showing more vaccine hesitancy than liberals. This polarization resulted in uneven impacts of the pandemic across different regions and communities, often correlating with political leanings. Thus, the pandemic challenged global health systems and laid bare the deep-seated political divisions within societies. The COVID-19 pandemic increasingly became a partisan issue rather than a unifying public health crisis.

The United States and Britain are not the only countries struggling with the political divide. Canada may be a prototype of patterns for other countries in the future. The French separatist movement has created significant political and cultural divisions within the country, concentrating national attention on the issue of Quebec's independence from Canada. This movement, driven by a desire to preserve French-Canadian culture and language, has overshadowed other political problems, as resources and political debates have been intensely focused on addressing the sovereignty question. The movement's push for independence has not only heightened tensions between Quebec and the rest of Canada but also within Quebec itself, as opinions on sovereignty vary among its residents. This internal focus on separatism has, at times, detracted from broader national discussions on other critical socioeconomic and political issues facing Canada as a whole.

The history of conservatism in Canada from 1945 to the present reflects a complex evolution marked by ideological shifts and the merging of conservative political entities. In the immediate post-World War II period, Canadian conservatism was primarily represented by the Progressive Conservative Party. This party, leaning toward traditional conservatism, emphasized the preservation of established institutions and a solid connection to the monarchy. Throughout the 20th century, Canadian conservatives often balanced between classic conservative principles and the need to adapt to a changing political landscape, including responding to the challenges of liberalism and social democracy.

Canadian conservatism underwent significant changes in the late 20th and early 21st centuries. The Progressive Conservative Party faced declining influence, leading to the emergence of new conservative factions, such as the Reform Party and the Canadian Alliance. These groups were more right leaning, focusing on fiscal conservatism, smaller government, and Western Canadian interests. The pivotal moment came in 2003 with the merger of the

Canadian Alliance and the Progressive Conservative Party, forming the modern Conservative Party of Canada. This merger signified a unification of various conservative strands in Canada, blending traditional Tory conservatism with the reformist and economically libertarian ideas of the newer conservative factions. Under leaders like Stephen Harper, the Conservative Party adapted to contemporary political issues, maintaining its relevance in Canadian politics.

In 2022, Canada was disrupted by the Freedom Convoy, an apparent grassroots movement from the politically conservative allied with truckers frustrated by the country's COVID-19 responses. This resulted in over 2,600 arrests and the brief occupation of downtown Ottawa. Canada may be heading toward the type of political discord that is now more common in the United States.

But Why Now?

Several factors have limited the feedback that has previously kept unfettered, unrealistic partisan growth restrained. In the past, personal contact and an ethic of human decency allowed compromise. This is often lacking in present-day social interaction which has shifted from in-person encounters to computer and phone screens. Second, standard media encouraged exposure to different viewpoints. With the advent of the internet, this is no longer common. Younger readers often fail to grasp how quickly this occurred. In their book "In the Year 2889" (1998), Jules Verne and his son imagined this change in how we would access information. This prediction came to fruition about 130 years later through various technological improvements (Thurman & Schifferes, 2012). Advances in predictive analytics and artificial intelligence, pioneered at first by Facebook but now ubiquitous, allow astounding predictions regarding what types of stories viewers will be interested in viewing. One key is the availability of vast amounts of data. One of the authors recalled when a colleague, a technology professor, demonstrated that social media sites could bypass traditional journalism vetting. "This may well be the end of democracy," she said.

As noted earlier, the rise of single-issue politics was the foundation for like-mindedness and echo chambers. Everything is amplified with no restraints, reflections, delays, or opposing viewpoints. "We've built a circuit without a single resistor. Not surprisingly, things heat up quickly and burn out." said an electrical engineer regarding single interest internet discussion groups.

In democratic countries like the United States, trust in social organizations and fellow humans is essential for a functional society. For many reasons, this trust has been decreasing for several generations. More recently, algorithms and isolation have encouraged even more distrust. Combined with individualistic tendencies, this may encourage many people to look to disinformation for information and direction. This results in an increase in isolation, toxic suspiciousness, and hostility that further fuels the basis of the "us against them" mentality.

Honorable Opponents to Mortal Enemies: The Process of Partisan Identity Formation

The divide between political factions polarizing large parts of our population is not new. What is different about democracies is that the transformation often involves the voluntary adoption of a specific ideology. People make choices that gradually influence and even dictate their worldviews. In the past, political adversaries could frequently be friendly or at least cordial and civil. Currently, with interactions marked by toxic distrust, this is much less likely..

The transition from amiable political adversaries to bitter enemies is a complex phenomenon shaped by many factors. Initially, individuals may engage in political discourse from differing but civil viewpoints. However, these differences can morph into deeply entrenched divisions as political polarization intensifies. The process often begins with confirmation bias, as people seek information that validates their beliefs, inadvertently isolating themselves from opposing perspectives. Obtaining reinforcement from people in their circle—the echo chamber—reifies their beliefs, quelling doubts.

Dehumanization is a pivotal stage in this transformation. As disagreements intensify, people may use derogatory language and stereotypes to describe their political adversaries, making it easier to vilify them. Media influence plays a significant role, as individuals consume news and commentary that further demonizes the opposing side, fueling negative perceptions. Social pressure within one's circles can also push people toward more adversarial stances, as they fear social consequences or ostracism for engaging with those from opposing political camps.

Emotions, such as anger and fear, can become dominant as conflicts escalate, eroding empathy for political adversaries. Personal identity can become deeply intertwined with political identity, making any challenge to one's beliefs feel like a personal attack. The process can ultimately culminate in outright conflict, including personal attacks or violence, as people become deeply entrenched in their positions. Families are fractured, couples fall apart, friendships are abandoned, and neighbors become estranged.

Mental health professionals in North America and elsewhere are still unlikely to encounter fully radicalized people seeking their help. It's most likely that this may happen for counselors and therapists who are working with involuntary clients. People who are court ordered into treatment, such as domestic violence or child abuse perpetrators, or those given ultimatums by employers or spouse are more likely to represent a broader range of political orientations. That is also the case with many people in treatment for addictive disorders who may have sought help under duress from employers or family members. Involuntary clients are essentially denied the ability to decline treatment under threat of legal penalties, divorce, or job loss. For clinicians working with these populations, there is more opportunity to work with people who would otherwise have avoided mental health treatment. Working with men and women ordered or coerced into treatment, clinicians learn to interact with clients who often harbor distrust of the mental health profession which is invaluable experience in working with politically polarized clients.

The Polarization Spectrum

We are currently in a situation where many moderate people have moved from reasonable to more extreme positions and beliefs. As mental health professionals, it is now likely that we will, sometime in our careers, treat individuals, couples, or families on the more extreme ends of the *polarization spectrum*. This is especially likely, as this chapter has discussed, because many people have been subjected to processes of mass political polarization. Jost, Baldassarri, and Druckman (2022) define mass political polarization as individuals becoming more politically divided or developing more intense group attachments. Ideological polarization is characterized as moving toward the extremes and away from the center concerning issues or ideology. Typically, this can result in a bipolar distribution, such as when a religious group discounts others. Partisan issue alignment occurs when groups divide over multiple issues, often because of differences in social factors. An example might be more classic splits on economic lines between working class and "country club" voters.

Affective polarization occurs when group members hold very high opinions of people from their group and very negative feelings toward those in other groups. These usually become self-reinforcing, further polarizing differences with outsiders. Affective polarization may offer social support, however, it has been linked with a variety of mental health effects, including anxiety and depression (Nelson, 2022). In each case, there is a separation, and it is well known in social psychology that the decisions of homogenous groups tend to be more extreme than those of individuals. In a later chapter, we will refer to this well-replicated phenomenon when we discuss depolarization.

Jost et al. (2022) propose psychological mechanisms that drive these polarization processes: ego justification, group justification, and individual differences and personal preferences. The first is the human tendency for ego justification, where people associate with people who endorse their views. We like others to believe what we believe and seek out those who support our views. This is increasingly common as we are more geographically and culturally separated.

Furthermore, we are all blinded by what social psychologists call the *ultimate attribution error*. Many people recall the fundamental attribution error, which focuses on attributions at the individual level. It refers to the tendency for people to underestimate situational factors and overestimate dispositional factors when explaining someone else's behavior. The ultimate attribution error deals with attributions at the group level. It refers to the tendency for groups to attribute positive ingroup behaviors to situational causes while attributing negative outgroup behaviors to dispositional flaws in the outgroup. When combined with the tendency to connect with others who endorse our views, we have a potent social tool for separating ourselves as good people and others as less desirable and flawed.

A second mechanism driving polarization is group justification, somewhat akin to the well-known process of cognitive dissonance. In group justification, people tend to justify the views of those with whom they affiliate. Religious groups have practiced this type of group justification and adherence for years. However, its common occurrence in politics has now become much more routine. For example, a person might not believe everything their radical organization endorses. Still, since the organization is essential to the person and the organization strongly endorses it, the person reasons that what the organization says must be somewhat accurate. Eventually, they come to believe it more fully, as people who have recovered from cult thinking can attest. We may not initially believe all of what our leader or party affiliates tell us, but in time, we will likely think more like them than we do now. We don't want to be rejected or alienated from those we've bonded with in the group.

A third mechanism driving polarization is related to individual differences and personal preferences identified in Chapter 2. Conservatives tend to identify with the status quo and may be more likely to resist change, pushing them together when social and individual changes are suggested. Liberals, on the other hand, tend to be more egalitarian, pushing them toward change around social issues or integrating them when crises occur. In either case, outside forces help people with diverse personalities coalesce into distinct groups composed of people similar to themselves. Once in these groups, they tend to be self-reinforcing, practicing group justification and ego justification, ultimately polarizing even further.

Understanding these mechanisms of polarization may help clinicians realize that the divide we're now witnessing is natural, not unusual or pathological. It may help the clinician understand their feelings and affiliation with their own "tribe" and how it has shifted. As Mason (2018) pointed out, identifying with a group because they are like us is simply a very human response, though one that can lead to severe political consequences.

Regardless of whether this is natural, some people are more likely to be highly partisan than others. Partisan thinking and behavior can dominate a person's interactions with others to the point where it can be considered socially toxic. While it may not be possible to "cure" the underlying structure that drives people to extremism, it may sometimes be possible to adjust the process of an individual on the trajectory. Different approaches to therapy may be most helpful depending on where the client's beliefs are in the spectrum of polarization.

A Model of Individual Partisanship for Counseling and Psychotherapy

As psychologists, we rarely find it necessary to impose a stages model on phenomena, except those related to biological or developmental issues. Stage models are often artificial. There is a genuine concern that the model may take on a life of its own. Some stage models, like the stages of grief, are assumed by many practitioners to be accurate even though many people do not fit into them, and there is minimal evidence to support them. Rigid stages imply a predictable and orderly progression, which is often untrue in real life. A similar model of political development would not necessarily be helpful. Human psychological and political development is incredibly complex and influenced by many factors, including personal experiences, cultural background, education, current realities, and socioeconomic status. Rigid developmental stages may oversimplify complexity by suggesting a linear or uniform progression everyone supposedly follows. Political beliefs can change, regress, or evolve in nonlinear ways. People might revisit certain beliefs or undergo radical changes due to significant life events or shifts in societal norms. Dynamic explanations allow for change and evolution over time, recognizing that political beliefs are not static but subject to change. They reflect a more realistic and human-centric view, acknowledging the possibility of stability and change.

Regardless, the stages we are proposing are heuristics. They are simplified and descriptive but not causal. However, they could help us understand the issues clients may need to discuss in counseling and therapy and may assist practitioners with the type of treatment they can offer when politics enters the therapy space. We have found the following five-stage model helpful in understanding this process. These are suggestions, not "ideal types" or even empirically based. Clinical observations may help organize the disparate data about political people. As models, they are maps, not the territory and there are many other ways to view this process.

Stage 1: The first stage of our partisan model can be considered the mildest stage of political identity and partisanship that may be troubling to others, including clinicians. It is where people become increasingly aware of the recognition of ideological division. They often exhibit strong divisions along ideological lines, with a deep commitment to the principles and policies of their political party or ideology (Pew Research Center, 2021). Identification at this stage is associated with the need for affiliation, acceptance, being understood, and belonging. People associate with people who are like them. They find acceptance, comfort, and affiliation. People hope to see or ultimately find meaning, which is a central life task, at least in Western cultures and those that emulate them. Typically, these are the passionate adherents found at political rallies, perhaps the people wearing t-shirts, political buttons, and yelling slogans. They may alienate their families somewhat and seem a bit opinionated. Still, their fervid enthusiasm is generally not out of line with traditions in a democratic country. People at this stage are often seen as a bit bullheaded and excessive. Still, they usually can understand when they need to separate their political beliefs from other aspects of social engagement. In other words, to quote a client, "I'm okay. I can turn it off if I have to."

Stage 2: The second proposed stage in the development of partisan ideology is a vehement increase in reaction toward opposing views. Exposure to highly partisan news or opinions from the other side often reinforces negative feelings toward political out-groups. This is usually accompanied by discordant knowledge (Gollwitzer, Olcaysoy Okten, Pizarro, & Oettingen, 2022). The more people are exposed to an idea counter to their beliefs, the more likely they will be convinced of the truth of their perspective and become more united in their group ideology. Exposure to ideas counter to their own may actually produce a visceral response; genuine anger or disgust.

Feelings of anger may follow an opponent process, a phenomenon long described by learning theorists, where exposure to a stimulus produces counter feelings. Trolling behavior, deliberately baiting political opposition with silly questions on the internet or elsewhere, may become common. Sometimes, these feelings can develop an addictive quality, as they can with a variety of opponent processes.

A liberal lawyer in a very conservative part of the country described her experiences being addicted to these counter feelings that she would generate when she was stressed.

> It was tough for me to live where I did. I didn't have a lot of support. Until I got into therapy, I would get on the internet, and I would go to various sites and just read the trash that the real nuts had written. It would just make me feel good about myself to start my day, or maybe during the day. It was just a sense of 'Thank God, my side is not that stupid.' That's a godawful way to get your sense of who you are, but it worked.

A Fundamentalist Christian pastor following an internet posting wrote:

> I used to get very upset when people would contradict scripture, you know social media things about the Flood being a myth and the like. Now, though, it's

like a gift. I go to read on the internet and there is no reason to refute it. I go, and I feel blessed reading what they write. I mean, I don't feel angry. I feel perfect.

We suspect that opponent processes may be involved. What may also be interesting is mocking, laughing, and belittling of opponent ideas or views. If done publicly or in internet space, these have the function of providing internal cohesiveness and helping a person bind with like-minded others. The more they mock and scoff at those who disagree with them, the more they identify with those who are like themselves. This leads to a natural third stage, where people and beliefs are attacked.

Stage 3: The third stage is associated with increased partisan antipathy or anger directed more specifically at people instead of ideas. There is a tendency for intense, sometimes personal, antipathy toward any members of the opposing political party or ideology. This can manifest in ascribing negative characteristics to those in the opposing party. Specific leaders may be especially mocked and scorned. Neither side has a monopoly on this type of thinking, which we have defined as *toxically partisanship*. It is in this stage where the development of racism, projective hostility, and group discrimination are likely to occur.

Stage 4: The fourth stage involves generating strong and irrational loyalty to a party, person, or concept. True believers demonstrate a strong adherence, dedication, or loyalty to their political party or a particular politician, often prioritizing party ideology over other considerations. It is in this stage that politicization can become cultlike. It was in this stage that average German citizens were transformed into their worship of the Fuhrer before and during World War II. During this stage, hyper-partisanship radicalization is possible (Bhui et al., 2019), a period where people will endorse truly bizarre beliefs because the party or the leader endorses them.

People don't need to have a specific leader for them to be caught up in this toxic process. For example, people associated with the "Q" phenomena were essentially leaderless. QAnon is a conspiracy theory that originated on internet forums in October 2017. It centers around an anonymous online figure or group of individuals known as "Q," who claim to have access to classified information within the U.S. government. The theory alleges that there is a secret plot against Donald Trump by a "deep state" group of Satan-worshipping pedophiles who are involved in a global child sex trafficking ring. The Tea Party arose in the early 2000s without a single leader and a single idea. Some adherents were partisan, while others were toxic. Similarly, some of the Black Lives Matter members in the United States held ideas that were exceptional, eccentric, and, by our definitions, toxic.

Stage 5: A fifth and final stage in the polarization process seems to involve internecine war among the faithful. People devoutly follow a philosophy, leader, or ideology and believe they are the true proponents or representation of it and actively seek to destroy those that follow similar teachings. As true believers narrow and fragment, almost every social psychological principle that operates to separate "us vs them" is magnified between the groups. For example, ideologies close to each other may see each other as a threat to their identity. When groups or individuals identify strongly with a particular ideology, they may feel that any deviation from it, even if slight, undermines the validity of their own beliefs.

Similar ideologies often compete for the same pool of supporters or adherents. This competition can lead to hostility as each group seeks to distinguish itself and prove its superiority. Furthermore, minor differences between closely related ideologies can be magnified and exaggerated, leading to heightened animosity. People may focus on these differences rather than the similarities, leading to increased polarization. For example, it's not enough to believe in the leader or philosophy, one must be ready to rise to violence against those who would silence them. Those who won't commit to that are not "true believers."

People who hold similar ideologies may reject compromise or cooperation with each other due to a belief that any concession dilutes their principles or legitimacy. This rejection can lead to further antagonism and hostility. At this stage, suspiciousness, paranoia, and fear dominate many social interactions.

Summary

Political divisiveness, while accentuated in recent times, is not a novel phenomenon but rather has deep historical precedents that span across cultures and epochs. This chapter explores the evolution of political polarization in America, highlighting the significant shifts from the 1960s onwards, where social movements and political events catalyzed a more pronounced ideological split. The analysis extends beyond the United States, examining similar patterns in the United Kingdom and other democracies, illustrating the global and complex nature of political polarization, which is shaped by a confluence of social, economic, cultural, and technological factors.

Further, the chapter offers an examination of the mechanisms and stages of partisan identity formation, illustrating how individuals can transition from moderate political engagement to extreme partisanship. It underscores the role of confirmation bias, social reinforcement, and emotional dynamics in deepening ideological divides, leading to a scenario where political identity becomes deeply intwined with personal identity. The discussion also touches upon the impact of modern communication technologies in amplifying these divides, creating echo chambers that reinforce and intensify partisan views. By dissecting the stages of partisan escalation, the chapter provides insights into the psychological and social processes that contribute to the transformation of political disagreements into deeply entrenched ideological battles, shedding light on the challenges and implications of navigating a highly polarized political landscape.

References

American Psychiatric Association. (1973). *Diagnostic and statistical manual of mental disorders* (2nd ed.). Washington, DC: American Psychiatric Association.

Bhui, K., Demunter, H., Dom, G., Frydecka, D., Gorwood, P., Kuey, L., Misiak, B., Raballo, A., Samochowiec, J., & Schouler-Ocak, M. (2019). A systematic review on the relationship between mental health, radicalization and mass violence. *European Psychiatry, 56*(1), 51–59. https://doi.org/10.1016/j.eurpsy.2018.11.005

Gollwitzer, A., Olcaysoy Okten, I., Pizarro, A. O., & Oettingen, G. (2022). Discordant knowing: A social cognitive structure underlying fanaticism. *Journal of Experimental Psychology: General, 151*(11), 2846.

Jost, J. T., Baldassarri, D. S., & Druckman, J. N. (2022, August). Cognitive-motivational mechanisms of political polarization in social-communicative contexts. *Nature Reviews Psychology*, 1. https://doi.org/10.1038/s44159-022-00093-5

Klein, E. (2020). *Why we're polarized*. New York: Avid Reader Press.

Mason, L. (2018). *Uncivil agreement: How politics became our identity*. Chicago: University of Chicago Press.

Nelson, M. H. (2022). Resentment is like drinking poison? The heterogeneous health effects of affective polarization. *Journal of Health & Social Behavior, 63*(4), 508–524. https://doi.org/10.1177/00221465221075311

Pew Research Center. (2021, November 9). *Beyond red vs. blue: The political typology*. www.pewresearch.org/topic/politics-policy/political-parties-polarization/political-typology/

Smith, K. B. (2022). Politics is making us sick: The negative impact of political engagement on public health during the Trump administration. *PLoS One, 17*(1), e0262022. https://doi.org/10.1371/journal.pone.0262022

Thurman, N., & Schifferes, S. (2012). The future of personalisation at news websites: Lessons from a longitudinal study. *Journalism Studies, 13*(5–6), 775–790. https://doi.org/10.1080/1461670x.2012.664341

Verne, J., & Verne, M. (1889). *In the year 2889.* Wildside Press.

4

THE QUESTION OF LIBERAL BIAS IN MENTAL HEALTH PROFESSIONALS

Mental Health Services Not Welcome: A View from the Frontline

On Sunday, June 5, 2022, the New York Times published a front-page story titled: "In Rural Town, Parents and Students Clash Over Mental Health" (Barry, 2022). Legislation to create school-based mental health clinics was overwhelmingly approved by the state lawmakers in Connecticut but "ran into a solid wall of resistance, mostly because it infringed on the rights of parents" (Barry, 2022, p. 21). While the article focused on Killingly, Connecticut, this story could have been about many towns in the United States.

School board meetings, which once focused on issues like approving budgets, adopting school calendars, and setting academic standards, have become stages for the political and social dramas that are typical of our contemporary news cycle. Even routine school board sessions can become a battleground for competing "culture wars" about various divisive topics, including mental health services. This clash over a proposal to offer mental health services at the local high school occurred between an elected school board and a small group of vocal parents. The divisiveness also took place between these parents and their high school-age children, most of whom favored the clinic. The school, the community, and many families were divided about how to best respond to the need for mental healthcare for students who were suffering from anxiety, depression, and other challenges to their mental and emotional well-being (Barry, 2022).

Why were these groups of parents saying that mental health services were not wanted in their school? Were they unaware of the increasing rates of mental health problems in young people? That is unlikely since the media reports this

DOI: 10.4324/9781032651217-4

trend quite frequently, and both the Left and Right use it for talking points. While the reasons for the increased mental health problems are complex and unclear, the increase is undeniable. Research conducted between 2016 and 2020 found that children and adolescents from ages 3 to 17 reported a 29% increase in anxiety in just four years. For depression, the rise was equally steep, at 27% (Brun-Harris, Chandour, Kogan, & Warren, 2022, July). One reason for the apparent sharp increase in mental health-related decline appears to be the COVID-19 pandemic. The increase in mental health problems during the first years of the pandemic was particularly evident for school-age children. As many parts of the country closed classrooms and transitioned to on-line teaching, children of all ages were missing out on the social and developmental benefits of being in a classroom. Parents attending the school board meeting to protest additional mental health resources in the school likely knew this information and certainly had direct experience of these challenges through their own children.

Why was there such opposition to providing additional mental health resources in schools to help mitigate these problems? On the surface, this does not seem to make sense. Are these parents somehow indifferent to their children's mental well-being? Are they in massive denial about the apparent indicators of depression, anxiety, anorexia, attention problems, autism, and learning disabilities that school counselors and psychologists were detecting? Don't they realize that mental health in children is essential for becoming well-functioning adults?

While we cannot truly know their motives, we believe that conservative parents are as committed to the health and welfare of their children as their liberal neighbors. It wasn't a lack of concern for their children. Instead, their reluctance was likely due to a deep-seated distrust of what the mental health profession represents. As one parent stated, "I do personally believe there's a lot of agendas out there ... and children are very malleable" (Barry, 2022, p. A1).

The parents protesting the availability of mental health services in the school felt that their values and beliefs were being undermined by bringing counselors into their schools who they perceived were trained in left-leaning academia. Many parents suspected that therapists who might work with their children would have more liberal views and would influence their children's thoughts in ways that were inconsistent with their family values and traditions. Another parent at the school board meeting believed that "... our modern-day psychology is rooted in occultism" (Barry, 2022, p. A21).

These parents, it seemed, feared that the mental health professionals would be advocating for more liberal values than their family held. They believed the effects on their families would be potentially problematic, perhaps even disruptive. This is a situation that family therapists have often seen when a closed, isolative system further self-insulates, blocking access to diverse ideas or information (Bütz, Chamberlain, & McCown, 1997). Unfortunately, this type of insulation is often unrecognized in individual therapy, where practitioners may forget that clients are part of a complex systems and receive feedback from many different sources including family members.

People who identify as conservatives typically prefer established traditions and are often less comfortable with novel approaches to resolving problems (Hibbing, Smith, & Alford, 2014). That is not a sign of psychopathology or instability but rather a different perspective regarding how to best solve problems in the family. Progressive or liberal therapists may see parents in these situations as uncaring, irresponsible, or worse. Conservative therapists may frame them instead as distrust of mental health professionals who do not share similar beliefs or world views and may be judgmental of their family's values.

Trying to find a therapist who shares or values a conservative viewpoint can often be challenging. Part of the problem may be that therapists feel awkward when the subject of politics arises. As a part of their clinical training, students learn to minimize self-disclosure, particularly about their cultural, religious, and political orientations. Counselors and therapists don't want to influence the client by introducing their own views, which clients may try to either emulate or reject. Traditionally, mental health professionals have been taught to avoid or downplay discussions of their own and their client's religious or political beliefs. These conversations are seen as too potentially biased and likely to create problems in the therapeutic alliance. Some approaches to psychotherapy and counseling view clients' political leanings as reflections of formative experiences in childhood or as ways to express anxieties. Regardless of a practitioner's theoretical orientation, however, mental health professionals are usually trained to avoid a direct conversation about a client's political beliefs other than reframing them as a reflection of unresolved conflicts or a part of their identity development.

It is not surprising that people with profound or highly charged political feelings assume that they cannot have an honest conversation with a counselor or therapist. They often feel left out, invalidated, awkward, constrained, and marginalized. They may fear being rejected or subjected to attempts to challenge or change their values and beliefs. Too often, the silence of well-meaning counselors makes matters worse.

A conservative client stated this feeling quite well:

A lot of Republicans I know who have tried counseling feel that they are being judged by leftwing therapists, kind of like we are not as good a person as them. If you voted for Trump and your counselor voted for anyone else, you know what I am talking about. You just feel they are looking down on you. It's worse if they won't talk about their political views. Their silence and the 'focusing on you, not me', it's really that they are judging us.

A very liberal university professor in a very conservative area noted the same feelings with opposite political dynamics:

> In the location where I live, most of the therapists, the doctors, accountants, just everyone is very conservative. But I am not. I do not hide it. I have been to several counselors for anxiety, which has been helpful, but the process has not been. It will come up that I don't own a gun or go to church. I don't believe in conspiracies. Whatever. Then, they get silent, like I am a cultural outcast. They don't know what to say, so they sink into this phrase I keep hearing over and over about not talking about politics. But they've already judged me and won't talk about it. Damn awkward!

Clients and Therapists: The Potential Political Mismatch

In the United States, about one-third more people identify as social conservatives than identify as liberals (Jones, 2023). Based on additional research (Appendix A), we estimate that about 45%–55% of clients seeking mental health treatment are politically moderate or more to the right. Most therapists, however, lean in a more liberal direction.. Approximately 60% of therapists in our sample identified as moderately liberal or progressive, and only 20% as conservative. Not so many mental health professionals are in the middle. In other words, there are probably three times as many liberal therapists as there are conservative therapists, and approximately half of people seeking mental health services identify as politically moderate or conservative.

How have we concluded that most therapists are more liberal than their clients? Aside from our research, other sources suggest that mental health professionals are far more likely to identify as liberals than as conservatives (Bilgrave & Deluty, 2002; Parikh, Post, & Flowers, 2011; Steele, Bischof, & Craig, 2014). For example, Norton and Tan (2019) note that over half of counselors and therapists describe themselves as "liberal," with less than a quarter of therapists who describe themselves as "conservative."

In some mental health professions, like Social Work, the number of liberal/progressive therapists probably outnumbers more conservative practitioners by a large percentage. Clinical Psychologists tend to be liberal leaning, at an estimated rate of three-to-one over more conservative clinicians. Psychiatrists also tend to lean left, though at a slightly lower rate. Marriage and Family Therapist (MFT) rates of liberal leaning practitioners are similar to psychologists, while licensed professional counselors are the most moderate but still more politically liberal than most of the population (Norton & Tan, 2019).

Maher (2021) makes a case that psychology and other mental health professions are predominantly liberal because their training emphasizes liberal values. For those of us with advanced degrees in psychology, social work, counseling, and related mental health fields, his statement accurately reflects the typical training experience. Also, a career as a mental health professional of any type is likely to attract more liberal-leaning students, those who are aligned with the moral foundations described by Jonathan Haidt (2012) as "Care" and "Fairness." The frequency of liberals in many areas of psychology was well documented recently by Frisby, Redding, O'Donohue, and Lilienfeld (2023). Liberals and progressives are the norm in both the clinical office and the classroom. While there are plenty of exceptions, they do not alter the base rate.

In interviewing conservative friends and associates, when asked whether they would seek psychotherapy if faced with a personal or relationship dilemma, they often voiced the concern that they would not be treated fairly and would be challenged to change their beliefs. These concerns are not categorically different from those described at the beginning of this chapter. For example, a woman whose marriage is based on a traditional foundation wherein the husband is responsible for making significant decisions and providing financial support for the family may fear being judged for her focus on being a wife and mother. Imagine that the woman is complaining about her husband's problem drinking. In that case, she might be framed as an "enabler" by addiction counselors, someone who is complicit in supporting her husband's alcohol use. She may be challenged by the therapist to confront or leave her spouse, two paths that may be antithetical to her beliefs.

A therapist's politics or worldview may not be initially apparent or might never be openly displayed. Still, mental health professionals are generally perceived by the public as leaning to the left. The simple knowledge that a psychologist, psychiatrist, counselor, or social worker has spent considerable time in academia pursuing their training and degrees is enough to place them in the "elitist" category for many right-leaning people. And, as noted, there's a good chance they are correct in that assumption. People who embrace solid conservative beliefs are more likely to encounter difficulty finding a therapist who has a deep understanding of their worldviews and even more difficulty finding someone who embraces and embodies those perspectives.

I was working with a married man whose wife discovered he was involved with using porn on-line. He was a deeply conservative person who sought help to 'save my marriage'. When I asked him if he wanted to find a couples' therapist and have sessions with his wife in addition to our individual work, he stated, 'I'm afraid that most counselors will tell her to leave me. Neither of us want that'.

(Social Worker, New York)

Therapists: Perhaps Not So Neutral

Therapists are generally trained to maintain neutrality; to be a "a blank slate." They believe that they are providing services in a value-free atmosphere, the way that many naïve people claim that they "do not see color." Perhaps this is the real difficulty. Unless a therapist is aware of their biases, they cannot monitor them and cannot realize how their perceptions may influence their world views and impact their relationships with clients. We know the risks of cultural insensitivity and bias with so many different populations yet fail to see this as important with clients whose political beliefs and values differ from ours.

Too often, clinicians are not aware that their clients hold different values nor how these values may affect their interactions in the therapy space. As discussed in Chapter 1, this division may be entirely natural. Given our justified emphasis on training in cultural competence, this ignorance on the part of therapists and counselors seems strange. To examine whether mental health professionals were aware of their biases, Chamberlain (2022) solicited responses from therapists on the *Better Help*™ therapist's forum, which is accessible to approximately 30,000 practicing therapists. *Better Help*™ is one of the most widely accessed teletherapy networks in the United States, and it has therapists and counselors throughout the country. This question was posted in an open discussion forum about responding to a client's statements regarding their political leanings: "I am interested in starting an ongoing conversation with providers about their experience providing services to members who have strong political/social issues beliefs. What has your experience been when those topics arise?"

Often, the results indicated either avoidance of the topic or denial that it was relevant. Common themes were articulated by therapists who responded anonymously.

> I focus on the underlying issues as they relate to the client's presenting issue and treatment plan. For example, unless they have come specifically to address an adjustment disorder related to elections or other politics-specific matters, it doesn't apply much. Just like with any other red herring, I lead the client back to the topic of most importance for their wellness.

Another therapist wrote:

> For me, those topics are just another opportunity to invite them to explore the unconscious part of their psyche that mostly drives human behavior.

And another noted:

> Politics is something that is part of a client's defenses and usually is a topic that serves to distract them from the real issues.

As illustrated through these responses, it is common for clinicians to try to either avoid political concerns or translate them into signs of some underlying disorder or unconscious dilemma. Sometimes, they project their issues onto their clients. The idea of a "red herring" was a common theme in response to political questions or inquiries. Yet paradoxically, almost all the therapists felt that political issues presented some challenges regarding how to work within the therapy relationship. Many of the therapists also stated that they were increasingly working with clients who were bringing in concerns related to political issues, such as abortion access, gun safety, and LGBTQ+ rights. The issue of conflict over politics in families and other relationships was also a topic that was more frequent on their list of presenting problems.

We believe that clients often want counselors and therapists to engage them regarding their stress associated with politics. Yet so often, therapists and counselors are unwilling, unable, or just too awkward about the topic to do so satisfactorily. Our professions haven't developed adequate training and guidelines to work effectively with the impact of political issues in our clients' lives.

Mental health professionals are trained to respect clients' autonomy. The goal is to remain neutral and open to any concerns that the client brings to therapy. How politics affects their lives is a topic that more clients want to discuss. Many of us find stepping outside our political orientations particularly challenging since they reflect our deeply held values. Due to the false consensus effect discussed earlier, therapists may question whether "sane" people can hold antithetical values to theirs. It may be difficult to appreciate that reasonable, mentally healthy people can see the world of social issues and politics from a very different perspective.

To manage this dissonance, some therapists refuse any conversations with patients that focus on political or social issues. Some others may, intentionally or not, use the therapy relationship to attempt to influence others to adopt their perspectives. Both positions are problematic, can undermine the therapy relationship, and potentially cause harm. Political beliefs have become increasingly woven into our lives. They are a salient factor in making choices about things like family planning, vaccinating our children, what version of news we consume, what books we approve for school libraries, how we view climate change, and whether we feel comfortable seeking help for psychological problems. We believe it is becoming impossible for a therapist to avoid these topics or act as though they don't matter in client's lives.

Most counselors and therapists try to stay balanced between political poles and focus on what *they believe* is essential to the client when they bring up political issues. However, clients may disagree. It's getting harder to fall back on a response like, "I'm neutral about those issues and am concerned about what they mean to you." That sleight of hand doesn't always work with clients with strong opinions and beliefs about political issues. Most clients know better; we're being evasive when confronted about our beliefs and values. While we don't want to change the focus during therapy sessions to ourselves and our thoughts, avoiding these topics can be equally damaging to the therapy relationship. Clients know that we're not a "blank slate" when it comes to our political beliefs and being disingenuous can impact one of the most important factors in a therapeutic relationship: trust.

Beyond this, a therapist's worldview affects how they classify their clients, respond to them, and react to them on an ongoing basis. Beliefs about social issues and religion are usually reflected in a person's political orientation and general worldview (Bilgrave & Deluty, 2002). It is simply not good therapy for a practitioner to be warm, supportive, and caring for most areas of a client's life and then suddenly become a neutral, blank slate without emotions or feedback when discussions turn to politics. Therapists are increasingly finding themselves questioned by clients who want to know about their positions on issues like abortion, transgender people, gun rights/safety, healthcare and medical information, and other topics that are flashpoints in our political climate.

We may question whether having a political opinion will bias our objectivity and other aspects of our ability to form a successful therapeutic connection. Currently, there are no specific studies regarding this for mental health professionals. There is research, however, from a study of primary care physicians that is relevant to understanding the influence of unrecognized political feelings. Hersh and Goldenberg (2016) examined how political orientation can influence patient assessment by presenting a variety of case vignettes to primary care physicians. Physicians were asked to rate the severity of hypothetical patients' problems, indicating how they would approach treatment. The results suggested that primary care physicians who were registered Republicans tended to focus on health risks associated with politically controversial behaviors identified by the Right as harmful, including marijuana use and abortion. They did this to a greater degree than their Democratic colleagues. They also noted differences in how Democrats and Republicans reacted to a vignette about guns in the home. Republican primary care physicians were more likely to focus on the safe storage of firearms. In contrast, their Democratic colleagues were more likely to discourage the patient from storing a firearm anywhere in the home.

A finding like this suggests that biases may influence several facets of treatment, especially when practitioners are unaware of them. We may ignore biases that appeal to our worldviews. Even the most progressive of us is quick to employ confirmatory biases. Reviews in the popular press and semi-scholarly areas, as well as the academic media tend to portray conservatives undesirably, with pejorative terms. One of the authors recalls reading popular psychology articles that labeled conservatives with language that, if applied to any other group, would be considered both highly offensive and irrational. An example is an article on the Psychology Today website titled: "Is Political Conservatism a Mild Form of Insanity?" (Schultz, 2008). There's concern about how many therapists felt smugly vindicated by these negative accounts as if their perceptions were finally proven true. Many of us probably felt the same reassurance about the other side when reading accounts in the popular press that support our own political biases. The need for justification is apparently so intense that it is reflected in multiple settings in both our intellectual and clinical lives.

Personal Political Biases Matter

Over many decades, research has focused on how racial, cultural, gender, and other biases in mental health providers have adversely affected mental health assessment, intervention, and treatment (Corrigan, 2004; Snowdon, 2003). It's been well established that biased provision of services is a barrier for historically marginalized populations (Merino, Adams, & Hall, 2018). Therapist-held biases can often engender empathic failures (clients don't "feel seen"), can cue feelings of invalidation, and increase an overall sense of mistrust, which can result in high attrition rates for clients. Low rates of voluntary engagement in therapy for specific populations are, at least in part, related to client's awareness that they may be misunderstood or even blamed for some aspects of their identity and life experience. People who have been historically marginalized or excluded in society are often correct in their suspicions that they will have similar experiences in psychotherapy (Corrigan, 2004). Education and training make current practitioners acutely aware of psychotherapy's potential for harm when we are unaware of our biases.

Historically, a lack of representation in the mental health profession of various racial, ethnic, cultural, religious, and other groups has been a significant deterrent to seeking help for many people. When it becomes challenging to find a therapist who understands your history, worldview, and value system, it can create a barrier to seeking help. Building trust can be challenging if someone seeks help from a therapist who is likely to embrace different values and perspectives. Maher (2020), a conservative therapist, described the concerns of people who had reached out to him for assistance in finding a therapist who would not be judgmental regarding their political views. He concluded that conservatives often view the mental health profession as filled with social justice activists who will judge them harshly for their values and will try to change their conservative views. They mainly feared being challenged to change their deeply held family traditions and religious values.

Psychotherapists, counselors, and all mental health workers must understand the political messages they may send clients through indicators in their work environment. Their political beliefs may make them blind to what the objects and symbols in their therapy space communicate to the clients. We send out signs of our values and beliefs in our offices, including our online workspaces; the books on the shelves, the items on our desks, and even what art is on the wall. We may not appreciate that these are signals that define our own choices or values, but to clients they have meanings that we completely miss. One of us recalls a highly conservative client who began to relax in cognitive behavioral therapy only when a contemporary abstract picture was removed from the therapy office and replaced with a pleasant-look, somewhat bland train poster, probably from the halcyon 1950s era. He said he was not aware of the artwork that had hung prominently. Yet his response was almost immediate and long-lasting. Apparently, the abstract art cued negative feelings for him because it was too progressive, while the train poster was more attuned to his values.

Liberal clients often respond to the use of gender-affirming pronouns (he/him, she/her, they/them, etc.) as necessary and as an important test of basic kindness and inclusion.. To many conservatives, though, the use of pronouns following one's name is both pretentious and a clear signal that the therapist or counselor is more liberal-leaning and potentially hostile to them. It is seen as "virtue-signaling," a shout-out to likeminded partisans. When working with clients where it truly matters, the use of proper pronouns is critical. More conservative clients, however, may see it as a "dog whistle," and sign that they may not be accepted by the counselor or therapist. It's important to know what we're communicating and what it indicates to those who are seeking our services.

Similarly, consider a 77-year-old conservative male veteran who completed an intake form in a mental health agency. He was offended by the cultural insensitivity of questions that the rest of us consider routine. "This asks me if I am a 'male,' 'female,' or 'other.' I don't even know what 'other' is? I didn't fight for my country to be asked if I was some 'other.'" The client then went on to accuse the therapist of being a "damn liberal," which, based on probabilities, was likely a correct guess.

While many mental health professionals may not recognize our left-leaning biases, often our clients may. This bias may also become more apparent if we step outside our roles and enter the legal system. In the United States, legal professionals tend to be more equally represented by lawyers and judges on both sides of the political spectrum. Those of us who have worked in the courts as examiners or expert witnesses expect to be challenged by allegations that we have a personal or political bias about specific social or legal issues (Edens et al., 2012). Accepting mental health expertise as neutral, accurate, and unbiased in a courtroom is the exception, not the rule. It's not only judges and lawyers who are often suspicious of mental health professionals' testimony; jurors may also view the expert as holding a liberal bias. Eden et al. (2012) found examples of disparaging comments about mental health experts as being partisan in 27% of the cases they reviewed. Given the increased political partisanship in the decade since this study, we might suspect that these perceptions of bias on the part of mental health experts in the legal system have risen.

To examine the presence of liberal bias in psychology and the social sciences, Haidt and colleagues created a questionnaire that measures people's scores on five moral foundations: Care, Fairness, Loyalty, Authority, and Sanctity (Graham, Nosek, & Haidt, 2012). The questionnaire can be accessed at https://yourmor als.org/. Readers are encouraged to take the questionnaire to provide a clearer sense of their values. Liberals and conservatives often respond differently to this questionnaire, a reflection of how we interpret and define the content of those moral foundations as described by Haidt (2012). People with a liberal bias tend to have the highest scores on the Care and Fairness foundations. In contrast, people with a conservative bias tend to score evenly on all five. Each group has different lenses through which they observe and interpret reality. This may certainly influence our work with clients.

The importance of cultural competency in training mental health professionals is well established. Indeed, an extraordinary number of people were mistreated, harmed, and irreparably damaged in the 19th and 20th centuries by the mental health field as it was developing. Overt and subtle racial discrimination, sexism, and other biases were as embedded in our approach to psychological issues and disorders as they were in other aspects of Western society at that time. We now acknowledge this reality and attest to its influence and legacy. For example, despite absolutely no empirical evidence, homosexuality was classified as a mental illness until 1973 (Dresher, 2015). It was also paradoxically criminalized in most jurisdictions around the world, ironic since it was also a diagnosable mental disorder. Women and minorities have historically been over-diagnosed and mistreated. In retrospect, the reasons for these attitudes look both self-serving and bizarre.

Since the 1980s, the importance of incorporating cultural competency into clinical training and professional development was increasingly embraced to reduce the harm being done to clients (Vasquez & Johnson, 2022). Training in all the mental health professions now requires courses focusing on understanding cultural differences and holding practitioners accountable for working in culturally sensitive and respectful ways with clients who are different from themselves. The pendulum was swinging toward increasing demands for fairness and justice, and rightly so. The individual's dignity was seen as necessary, if not paramount, to establishing an effective, respectful therapeutic alliance. Therapist self-awareness and cultural humility is now much more normative regarding ethnic, gender, and racial issues (Harris et al., 2024)

Some mental health professionals now suggest that problems have existed in how we have omitted conservative clients from our understanding of culture. Social justice ideology and promoting social activism as a part of being a mental health professional have become more embedded in therapist training. The American Counseling Association (ACA), National Association of Social Workers (NASW), and American Psychological Association (APA) have all included statements in their core professional values that emphasize the importance of social justice as a part of professional competency. We're encouraged, and with good reason, to advocate for fair and equal treatment and services for groups who have been the focus of discrimination, oppression, unfair treatment, or exclusion from full participation in our society.

Yet for mental health professionals who are more conservative leaning, there is a rising concern about the division of people into "oppressed" and "oppressors." They question this labeling of people based on their racial, cultural, gender, sexual, and political identities and believe this leads to assumptions that can inhibit productive work in therapy. Indeed, that was the case in the past for women, people of color, LGBTQ+ individuals, and culturally or religiously diverse people. Now, the concern is for those who are being described as "oppressors," particularly males, white people, Judeo-Christians, and conservatives.

Mental health professionals must always realize that exploitation and victimization is real, both historically and currently. It continues today and can occur in unlikely places. But often our stereotypes blind us to its existence. One of the authors recalls classes as a professor at a rural college in a conservative area, where many female students (who usually comprised 80% to 90% of the class) clearly stated that they would not feel comfortable working with men in counseling. For many this was based on histories of abuse or violence in their relationships. Other women felt male clients would sexualize or oppress them in counseling relationships. These were largely "traditional," right-leaning women, yet their fears were based on their life experiences and often there was no one that they could confide in regarding their feelings. Using language associated with victimization, categories popular among left-leaning therapists, would have been both offensive to them and would have failed to acknowledge the realities and victories of their life struggles. These women would be unlikely to describe themselves as "victims" or part of an oppressed group. Instead, they wanted skills to deal with obstacles to their life goals.

Invoking labels of "oppressor" or "male patriarchy" or other shibboleths might well have been the easy way out. Instead, the focus was on the students' feelings and helping them develop viable plans for working where they felt the most comfortable. The instructor never denied the reality of the students' feelings and encouraged them to explore their experiences to the extent they felt comfortable. The students were not pressured or required to develop narratives that were not their own.

On many college/university campuses in North American and Europe there is likely to be a bias toward the left. While some of this may be due to younger people typically being more liberal, college faculty also tend to be politically more progressive than the general population, particularly in the social sciences. Shields and Dunn (2016) surveyed professors in the United States regarding their political leanings. They assessed that only 9% identified with the conservative party (Republicans). In psychology departments, an even higher ratio of educators identified as liberal: 10.5 liberal professors to 1 conservative professor (Duarte et al., 2015). Since every mental health professional, whether a psychiatrist, counselor, social worker, nurse, psychologist, or pastoral counselor, takes psychology classes, the likelihood of taking courses from liberal leaning professors in the United States is exceptionally high. The combined milieu and values of a university, along with social pressures and the shame of having different ideas, may have a substantial impact on college age students, directing them to think less critically about liberal ideas. It may also be a challenging experience for people who hold conservative viewpoints and may fear being excluded and ostracized.

Throughout our professional training, we are challenged to expand our awareness and understanding of dilemmas faced by the clients we encounter. Undergraduate and graduate programs in psychology, social work, and human services require classes that focus on increasing our knowledge, understanding, and compassion to serve a wider variety of our fellow citizens. We train ourselves to be more aware of histories of oppression, discrimination, stigma, prejudice, and other factors that continue to be experienced by many in our country. We learn about different cultural and religious practices and explore how our clients are influenced by these essential aspects of their lives and histories. Training ourselves to recognize and acknowledge our own experiences and histories and the biases we carry helps ensure that we don't judge or pathologize clients with different histories, identities, and life experiences. It is critical to all who seek our services to feel understood and accepted, even conservatives! Establishing and maintaining a trusting, effective therapeutic relationship with someone means we respect and appreciate the values and experiences they bring to our work together.

Should There Be a Political Divide Among Therapists?

In the mental health field, it's common to let clients know if we have an affinity for working with specific clients. For example, some professionals note special expertise or comfort with religious issues (Christian counselors) or sexual/gender concerns (LGBTQ+ counselors). Perhaps, for those who acknowledge their political leanings, it may be worthwhile to consider adding that information to our list of affiliations. For example, at Better Help™, a teletherapy service, when new clients are searching for a therapist who matches their preferences, they can indicate that they want a "liberal" or "conservative" therapist if that is important to them. This allows them to have some sense of being matched with a therapist who is less likely to react negatively to their worldviews.

Conversely, others argue that counseling and psychotherapy should not be bifurcated between two polarities of political extremes. They maintain that mental health professionals should not advocate for a split between practitioners who primarily treat people on the right and another group more comfortable with liberals. However, as Maher (2020) notes, "Political inclusivity is not a strength of the mental health profession." The public perception of liberalism in our field has implications for who will and won't seek out our services. Conservative clients may understandably be less likely to seek assistance from mental health professionals if they think that their political beliefs could become a central issue in their therapy. The fear of being stigmatized or persecuted can be a crucial factor in deciding whether to seek help or continue to suffer from a psychological problem (Silander, Geczy, Marks, & Mather, 2020). This creates a barrier for many people who may benefit from counseling services but want to avoid being stigmatized or judged by their therapist. It's a similar pattern that we've seen with many other populations who haven't seen themselves represented by professionals in the mental health field.

Therapists who hold more conservative beliefs are now stepping forward and addressing the disparity in the availability of right-leaning professionals. As an example, a web page and blog established by a conservative therapist is reaching out to people on the right who may be seeking mental health services. Their "Conservative Therapists" information page (www.conservativetherapists.com/) begins with the following statement:

> Some Conservative Americans in this polarized era are looking for a therapist, psychiatrist, or healer who either has the same values or who is affirming and open-minded to a Conservative belief system. This makes perfect sense to me, especially because many Liberal therapists do not have unconditional positive regard for Conservatives.
>
> *(Conservative Therapists, 2023)*

Another resource is the Open Therapy Institute (OTI) which addresses issues in mental health that are overlooked as a result of sociopolitical bias. The OTI provides both training workshops and research opportunities to therapists interested in learning more about the interface between therapy and politics. They also offer referrals to qualified therapists who are dedicated to working with clients with diverse, conservative-leaning values. In their introduction to the Institute, they state the following:

> Not long ago, there was a consensus in the mental health field that therapy should be client-centered. It was seen as unethical for therapists to impose political ideologies on sessions or to judge or reject clients for their political views. Therapists were encouraged to think empathically toward all of their clients, whatever their beliefs. Sadly, this consensus is now being replaced by approaches that prioritize political ideology over quality care. This change is leaving many people without good options.
>
> As therapy becomes more politicized, many people are reasonably concerned about therapists' biases interfering with their treatment. More and more people feel stifled, including centrists, moderates, libertarians, and many liberals, as well as people who are just open-minded. Now, many of these people are having a harder time finding a therapist who is truly open to their values and experiences.
>
> *(Open Therapy Institute, 2024, www.opentherapyinstitute.org)*

Davis (2023), in an article titled "How Therapists Became Social Justice Warriors," described conversations with therapists and clients who were negatively affected by the intrusion of "identity politics," which often ascribes categories like "victim" or "oppressor" to clients based on traits like their race, gender, and political identification. She expressed alarm that the professional who was supposed to help ease her trauma became an additional source of it when therapy sessions focused on ideology rather than the circumstances that she experienced (Davis, 2023).

There may be problems that are so culturally challenging that liberal or progressive therapists cannot be comfortable with working with certain clients. A colleague of one of the authors shared her dilemma of trying to work with woman who became pregnant following a rape and wanted to keep the child due to her religious and culturally beliefs. She couldn't see this as an acceptable choice. She was unable help the client process what had happened and support her decision to keep the child and prepare to be a loving parent. We may lack sufficient cultural competence to address some issues. This is recognized in other areas. For example, therapists or counselors who lack understanding of a specific cultural aspect of their client will often attempt to refer the client to someone who has a greater familiarity of factors relevant to a client's needs. Concerns occur when therapists lack the experience or wisdom to make these referrals or when they simply have no resources. At that point, constant self-awareness is necessary to prohibit the therapist or counselor from inadvertently attempting to impose their values in the therapy space.

How One Therapist Handles the Divide

Paul Norris, a MFT in San Francisco, has the following statement on his practice webpage that speaks to the idea of being more thoughtful about ideological balance. On his information page, "Therapy with Paul: Therapy and Politics," he states the following:

> The place of politics in therapy is far from being an easy topic. Many therapists refuse to allow clients to speak of politics at all. Others consider this area to be best avoided. Some think it legitimate to push clients toward the therapist's political orientation, somehow convincing themselves that this is in the client's best interest. Every time I hear this from a friend or potential client, I am deeply saddened. Interestingly, I have not heard therapists themselves proclaiming that this is what they do. In my view, doing so violates the sacred trust at the heart of therapy.
>
> I think anything that causes suffering in our lives has a place in the context of therapy. It's also clear that people's political orientation can be very core to their sense of self, and my job is to respect their choices. This is my approach in both individual and couple's therapy. In my practice, well-being and relationships are the priority.
>
> Should you choose to work with me and bring up political choices and beliefs, I will handle this area in the same way that I handle all others. I will work within the scope in which you give me permission. We can investigate how choices you make are helpful or detrimental to your sense of well-being. Thus, I will not challenge whether you are left, right or other. If you are open to it, I will work with you to look at how you express or follow your beliefs, and whether that is working for you. This may or may not include how you use social media, how much time you spend consuming news, and what sources you choose.
>
> Alternatively, you may just want someone who will listen in an open-hearted way to what you experience. If you wish, I will give you my complete support in this choice.
>
> *(Norris, 2023)*

We believe this is a nicely balanced statement about what clients can expect if or when they want to share something in therapy regarding their experiences with social and political issues or ideology. It's respectful of clients across the political spectrum and clearly states a position of openness to hearing any concerns they may have about the impact of politics on their lives. The statement also addresses anxiety the client might have about being judged negatively by the therapist for their beliefs. It informs clients that they can explore the impact of politics on their lives if that is a salient issue for them. It also acknowledges that clients are more likely to raise issues related to social issues and politics than might have been the case historically and opens this area for work in the therapy space.

Summary

A frequently overlooked bias is the tendency of mental health professionals to lean to the left of the political spectrum. Many right-leaning citizens know the bias is there; now it's time for us in the helping professions to acknowledge and address this dilemma. We believe it's as essential for us to be aware of how our politics and worldview influence us as it is to recognize the other forces that influence us such as our culture, religion, race, and gender. Personal biases, particularly those we haven't acknowledged, continue to influence how we work with people despite training and coursework to improve our self-awareness and to better understand and appreciate diverse populations.

References

Barry, E. (2022, June 5). In rural town, parents and students clash over mental health. New York Times (pp. A1, A21).

Bilgrave, D. P., & Deluty, R. H. (2002). Religious beliefs and political ideologies as predictors of psychotherapeutic orientations of clinical and counseling psychologists. *Psychotherapy: Theory, Research, Practice, Training, 39*, 245–260. https://doi.org/10.1037/0033-3204.39.3.245

Brun-Harris, L. A., Chandour, R. M., Kogan, M. D., & Warren, M. D. (2022, July). Five-year trends in US children's health and well-being, 2016–2020. *JAMA Pediatrics, 176*(7).

Bütz, M. R., Chamberlain, L. L., & McCown, W. G. (1997). *Strange attractors: Chaos, complexity, and the art of family therapy.* New York, NY: John Wiley & Sons.

Chamberlain, L. (2022, May). *On-line survey of better help psychotherapy providers.*

Conservative Therapists. (2023, March 12). *Conservative therapists: Why we exist.* www.conservativetherapists.com/

Corrigan, P. (2004). How stigma interferes with mental health care. *American Psychologist, 59*, 614–625.

Davis, L. (2023, May 17). *How therapists became social justice warriors.* www.thefp.com/p/how-therapists-became-social-justice-warriors?

Dresher. (2015, December 4). Out of DSM: Depathologizing homosexuality. *Behavioral Science, 5*(4), 565–575.

Duarte, J. L., Crawford, J. T., Stern, C., Haidt, J., Jussim, L., & Tetlock, P. E. (2015). Political diversity will improve social psychological science. *Behavioral and Brain Sciences, 38*, 1–58.

Edens, J. F., Smith, S. T., Magyar, M. S., Mullen, K., Pitta, A., & Petrila, J. (2012). "Hired guns," "Charlatans," and their "Voodoo Psychobabble": Case law references to various forms of perceived bias among mental health expert witnesses. *American Psychological Association, Psychological Services, 9*(1), 259–271.

Frisby, C. L., Redding, R. E., O'Donohue, W. T., & Lilienfeld, S. O. (Eds.) (2023). *Ideological and political bias in psychology: Nature, scope and solutions.* Cham, Switzerland: Springer.

Graham, J., Nosek, B., & Haidt, J. (2012). The moral stereotypes of liberals and conservatives: Exaggeration of differences across the political spectrum. *PLoS One,* *7*(12). https://doi.org/10.1371/journal.pone.0050092

Haidt, J. (2012). *The righteous mind: Why good people are divided by politics and religion.* New York, NY: Vintage.

Harris, J., Jin, J., Hoffman, S., Phan, S., Prout, T. A., Rousmaniere, T., & Vaz, A. (2024). *Deliberate practice in multicultural therapy.* Washington, DC: American Psychological Association.

Hersh, E. D., & Goldenberg, M. N. (2016). Democratic and Republican physicians provide different care on politicized health issues. http://hdl.handle.net/10079/40ff5 2f4-19e2-417c-9df3-4df32ae59f62, ISPS Data Archive

Hibbing, J. R., Smith, K. B., & Alford, J. R. (2014). *Predisposed: Liberals, conservatives, and the biology of political differences.* New York, NY: Routledge.

Jones, J. M. (2023, June 8). *Social conservatism in the U.S. highest in about a decade.* Gallup, Inc. https://news.gallup.com/poll/506765/social-conservatism-highest-dec ade.aspx

Maher, R. D. (2020, July 16). *Conservative psychologist wanted.* www.psychologyto day.com

Maher, R. D. (2021, August 20). *The therapist's dilemma: Political neutrality or disclosure?* www.psychologytoday.com/us/blog/the-conservative-social-psycholog ist/202108/the-therapists-dilemma-political-neutrality-or?eml

Merino, Y., Adams, L., & Hall, W. (2018, June). Implicit bias and mental health professionals: Priorities and directions for research. *Psychiatric Services, 69*(6), 723–725.

Norris, P. (2023). *Therapy with Paul: Therapy and politics.* Retrieved May 1, 2023, from https://paulenorris.com/index.php/therapy-and-politics/

Norton, A. L., & Tan, T. X. (2019). The relationship between licensed mental health counselors' political ideology and counseling theory preference. *American Journal of Orthopsychiatry, 89*(1), 86–93.

Open Therapy Institute. (2024). www.opentherapyinstitute.org/

Parikh, S. B., Post, P., & Flowers, C. (2011). Relationship between a belief in a just world and social justice advocacy attitudes of school counselors. *Counseling and Values, 56*(1–2), 57–72. https://doi.org/10.1002/j.2161-007X.2011.tb01031.x

Schultz, W. T. (2008, September 6). Is political conservatism a mild form of insanity? *Psychology Today.* www.psychologytoday.com/us/blog/genius-and-madness/200809/ is-political-conservatism-a-mild-form-of-insanity

Shields, J. A., & Dunn, J. M. (2016). *Passing on the right: Conservative professors in the progressive university.* New York, NY: Oxford University Press.

Silander, N. C., Geczy, B., Marks, O., & Mather, R. D. (2020). Implications of ideological bias in social psychology on clinical practice. *Clinical Psychology: Science and Practice, 27*(2).

Snowdon, L. R. (2003). Bias in mental health assessment and intervention: Theory and evidence. *American Journal of Public Health, 93,* 239–243.

Steele, J. M., Bischof, G. H., & Craig, S. E. (2014). Political ideology and perceptions of social justice advocacy among members of the American Counseling Association. *International Journal for the Advancement of Counseling, 36*(22), 450–467. https://doi.org/10.1007/s10447-014-9217-0

Vasquez, M. J. T., & Johnson, J. D. (2022). *Multicultural therapy: A practice imperative.* Washington, DC: American Psychological Association. https://doi.org/10.1037/0000279-000

5

POLITICS INVADES
THE THERAPY SPACE

The Therapist's Phone Rang …

It was likely just a routine call for an appointment. The speaker slowly identified himself as reluctant to make a new therapeutic contact. He was 34. He was Caucasian and worked as a parts supply manager. He had recently undergone a lingering, unpleasant breakup with his longtime girlfriend. He said that he was now having trouble sleeping. Furthermore, he was preoccupied with this past relationship. He spent too much time looking at old videos of his previous partner and him together that seemed to pop up without warning on his phone.

He said reluctantly that he drank too much whiskey and often bet excessively on the NFL and college games. He was smoking too much weed. He had even texted an old friend who volunteered that he "knew someone" who could get him opiate pills "to take the pain off the breakup." By his account, he was losing control.

His brother, with whom he now lived, said he was worried. While recounting this, the prospective client opened up a bit. "My brother says I've never been quite this depressed. Not since our grandfather died. He said I-he's afraid I might do something that winds up … yeah, hurting me. On bad days, maybe he is right." When asked if this was true, the respondent slowly said, "Not yet". He denied a suicidal plan. "But I don't know who I am kidding. I guess I could get there if I didn't get help. Soon."

He was particularly bothered that good friends told him to ignore his feelings. "They are telling me, 'Get drunk. Just go out. You just need to meet someone new. Find someone to hook up with. Whatever. Just stop looking at

DOI: 10.4324/9781032651217-5

all those old videos. Quit social media. Just get over her.' Some days, I think I am making progress. Some days, I just feel so stupid."

His primary medical provider, a nurse practitioner, was savvier than his friends. Without being told, she believed something deeper might be wrong. She recommended that he talk to a counselor or therapist before his life spiraled out of control. "So that's why I called. A friend of mine went to see you when her kids were having trouble. She said you were, well, 'very good with feelings.' She said you were easy to talk to, not judgmental. Also, she said you really helped her family. I was wondering .... Could you see me sometime? The sooner, the better, I guess."

Following a few questions, the therapist concluded that the new client was not in immediate danger. He explained the intake procedure, fees, insurance options, appointment times, and limits of confidentiality. Then he explained how therapy works, how long it would take, the degree of motivation involved, and the issues it might address. The new client seemed optimistic. With a minimal delay, he agreed to an appointment in two days.

The client made one final comment while going over directions to the therapist's office. "I want to make sure of one thing if that is okay. One thing before I see you. It is kind of weird but important. To me, at least." The therapist agreed, thinking it would be a question about confidentiality, training, insurance, or even dual relationships. But he was wrong.

"Tell me", the client said agitatedly, "and this may be weird, but it is important to me. Who did you vote for? I mean for President. I hate to ask because it's a free country and all, but I don't think I could trust some 'Snowflake' who thinks I am some kind of closet 'Deplorable.'"

The therapist was unsure how to respond. It seemed like such a violation of the therapy space.

What Is the Therapy Space?

The therapy space refers to a concept embraced by counselors and therapists to describe not just the physical setting of counseling and psychotherapy but also the emotional atmosphere of the therapeutic environment (Chamberlain, 2021). Typically, physical aspects, such as the room's layout, lighting, and decor, are chosen to make clients feel at ease and creates a place where they can engage in the therapeutic process without external distractions or judgments. But beyond the tangible elements, the therapy space embodies a psychological and emotional atmosphere characterized by respect, empathy, understanding, and a nonjudgmental stance from the therapist. This environment fosters the therapeutic alliance—a collaborative and trusting relationship between the therapist and the client. The therapy space is a cornerstone of effective therapy, providing the emotional safety needed for clients to explore their inner worlds, confront challenging issues, and embark on a journey of self-discovery and healing.

The positive use of the therapy space lies in its ability to facilitate open communication, emotional processing, and self-reflection. Clients are encouraged to voice their experiences and emotions within this space, supported by the therapist's guidance. This process allows for a deeper understanding of oneself, leading to insights into personal behavior patterns, relationship dynamics, and emotional responses. The therapy space thus becomes a catalyst for change, enabling clients to work through difficulties and move toward personal growth and resolution. This is true regardless of the counselor or therapist's training, their theoretical or treatment orientation, and whether they are providing therapy in an office setting or online.

As mental health professionals have learned from teletherapy, the therapy space transcends the physical confines of a room, embodying an environment where healing and transformation are nurtured. Therapists empower their clients to navigate the complexities of their emotions and experiences by creating a safe, empathetic, and understanding environment. This carefully cultivated space is crucial for the therapeutic process, offering a foundation for clients to achieve the change and well-being they seek.

Counselors and therapists typically attempt to keep politics and political topics out of the therapy space, and generally, their intentions are good. They desire to maintain a comfortable environment so that the focus is on the client's inner experiences and personal growth. In other words, they want to make sure that the therapeutic alliance is not compromised by things that might distract or agitate the client. The perception of a therapeutic alliance is one of the most critical factors in psychotherapy outcomes (Cuijpers et al., 2019). Political discussions in sessions can risk compromising the therapist's neutrality and, hence, this alliance. When therapists bring their own political biases into the therapy room, this can damage objectivity and impair their ability to serve the client (Farber, 2018).

Additionally, political views are deeply rooted in people's identities and values. Disagreements over political problems between therapist and client can fracture the trusting therapeutic alliance they need to make progress. Like religion, politics can be a divisive issue that could create a breach of trust in the therapeutic relationship if our political views differ significantly from the client's. The therapy space is designed to help clients gain insight into themselves, unpack complex emotions, and make positive changes through self-understanding. Getting embroiled in political debates and controversies can distract from focusing on the inner work clients need to do to reach their goals. The therapy space may be the only chance for people to define themselves and express their narratives without judgment and biased interference.

For therapy to be effective, clients must feel safe candidly expressing their thoughts, feelings, and struggles without fear of judgment or rejection. Discussing today's often polarizing political issues may lead clients to censor themselves or worry about being negatively perceived for their beliefs and opinions. This could create an unsafe emotional climate that inhibits openness and vulnerability. Politics and political events can also trigger strong emotions like anger, anxiety, grief, and hopelessness for clients. Best practices have always assumed that keeping politics out of the therapy space preserves objectivity. The purpose of the therapy space is to provide a haven that avoids divisiveness, maintains focus on personal growth, and ensures emotional safety. Avoiding politics, like avoiding discussions about religion, can prevent triggering vulnerable clients. Avoidance may, however, inhibit clients from exploring issues or experiences that contribute to their mental, emotional, and/or relationship distress. The intention is to provide the best care possible to facilitate clients' healing and development. These practices are now being challenged by political polarization.

Politics and the Therapy Space

Maintaining the neutrality of the therapy space has become increasingly difficult in recent times. One reason is simply that clients are often distracted by the constant clamor and animosity of our politics. They hear about politics, read about political events, are asked about politics, and are dominated by a cycle of political grabs for their attention. Not surprisingly, this badgering cycle of overexposure can take its emotional toll (Panagopoulos & Weinschenk, 2023). Relationships with family, friends, coworkers, and neighbors are strained over constant, sometimes petty, political disagreements. People feel angry, afraid, and anxious about the uncertainty of political issues and the impact on their lives. These distractions make it more difficult for clients to engage in introspection and achieve whatever goals they are attempting to pursue in therapy.

Beyond distraction, the current heated political climate is also a significant source of chronic stress for many Americans and people elsewhere. Research shows consistent exposure to political tensions increases risks for anxiety, depression, poor sleep, emotional outbursts, obsessive thoughts, and strained relationships. Smith (2022) estimates that between a fifth and a third of adults in the United States, approximately 50 to 85 million people, blame politics as the primary factor in fatigue, sleep disturbances, loss of control of anger, and triggering impulsive or compulsive behaviors (e.g., posting negative comments on social media that they later regretted; perseverating about political issues). Approximately 40%—more than 100 million—consistently identify politics as a significant source of stress. A study by Ford, Feinberg, Lassetter, Thai, and

Gatchpazian (2023) suggested that politics can be a daily, chronic stressor, decreasing feelings of well-being. An article in the American Psychologist noted, "Modern politics—its daily controversies, incivility, and ineptitude—puts a regular emotional burden on Americans" (APA, 2023). The constant political upheavals affect even apolitical, politically independent, and politically moderate individuals.

Political stress affects conservatives and liberals alike. Often, those of us who are left-leaning believe we are the only group that feels stress from politics. Yet both sides feel the tension. In the United States, liberal-leaning people may not realize that conservatives may think that *they* do not have freedom of speech; in more liberal states in the United States, conservative-leaning residents may feel isolated, just as liberals in more conservative areas may feel alone and fearful. Across the political spectrum, uncertainty about the nation's future causes significant unease regardless of a person's politics.

As most clinicians realize, psychotherapists have generally been cautioned to avoid discussions about politics in the therapy space (Birbilis, 2018). Although mental health professionals are trained to engage across cultures and work with clients from different backgrounds and social experiences, we rarely encounter training to help us work across the political spectrum. Solomonov and Barber (2019) note: "This is quite surprising given the significant effect of the political climate on patients' and therapists' everyday lives" (p. 1509).

The first quarter of the 21st century has led to clients with new types of problems within the therapy space. "Patients seeking psychotherapy for the first time are often more vulnerable than they have ever been in their adult lives" (Kindsvatter, 2024). These are people who enter therapy because they are considering major or irrevocable life decisions that are related to political concerns or stress. There are many examples of the types of stressors that cause their behaviors. Parents cite climate change as influencing family planning. In an international survey (1,000 parents each in the United States, India, Mexico, Singapore, and the United Kingdom), more than half of parents in each country reported climate change as a critical aspect of their decision to have children. Ninety-one percent of those surveyed shared that they were specifically concerned about rising temperatures, water shortages, sea levels changing, and significant weather events like hurricanes or floods (Lee, Ashton, Griep, & Edmonds, 2018).

Recently, one of the authors has worked with several married women whose presenting problem was anxiety about starting a family. They were worried about bringing a child into a world that they believe is becoming more inhospitable to life as we know it. They questioned what type of future their child would inherit and the quality of life they would have. This concern was not a "red herring" or a symbolic reflection of some unconscious or internal dynamic; they were worried about what life would be like for a child they brought into a world undergoing significant changes. These women were struggling, along with their partners, about whether they were making a responsible, moral choice regarding both their potential child's future and the future of the planet.

Individuals and families on both sides of the divide are taking the "extraordinary step of moving to escape a political or social climate they abhor" and relocating to other states that more closely align with their political leanings (Gabriel, 2023). Neighborhoods are becoming more segregated by political affiliation, and there are increasing reports of people moving to different areas of the country that align with their political values. A quarter of Americans have seriously considered moving because of politics. Counselors and therapists may fail their clients if they do not understand that clients need support when considering these difficult decisions. Avoiding these charged topics compromises our ability to assist clients in times of crisis.

Politics and political fears may also disproportionately affect people with historical legacies of disenfranchisement. For example, LGBTQ+ youth suffer increased anxiety and depression amid legislation restricting their rights. For younger people, specific legislation can have a significant impact on their mental health that older people often overlook. Research shows an increased risk of suicide and poor mental health for LGBTQ+ individuals in states that have passed restrictive bills (Novotney, 2023). Nearly two in three LGBTQ+ young people report an increase in anxiety and depression when hearing about potential state or local legislation that would prohibit discussions about LGBTQ+ people in schools. In the United States, bills that aim at eliminating programs for diversity, equity, and inclusiveness may be seen as triggering remembrance of racist feelings or as harbingers of future activities. Protests about the Israeli/Gaza war are seen as antisemitic and trigger Holocaust fears.

Following the Supreme Court's decision to overturn Roe v. Wade, I met with clients who were deeply affected by this decision. Several clients came into therapy precisely because they were concerned about this change. They wanted to share their thoughts and reactions and discuss how this court ruling significantly affected them. Not only was the Court's decision a factor, but many were affected by the changes in legislation in their home states and by some of the rhetoric that supported those decisions. I worked both with clients who felt devastated and angry about the change and clients who expressed relief and appreciation that abortion was no longer as accessible as it once was. It certainly was not a topic that I could avoid or ignore, and it brought the client's political leanings into the foreground of our work.

(a female psychologist in Florida)

In the Deep South and other conservative areas, it is not uncommon for people to come into therapy regarding abortion, but from a different perspective. A therapist colleague recalled a client who came into therapy to discuss her sister, who was a 'health-care' professional but who had multiple abortions. The client felt guilt over this – vicarious guilt over her sister's choices. Supporters of the right to choose may find this difficult to consider or respond to in therapy. Other clients will seek counseling or therapy many years following an abortion and have lingering doubts. In the South, this may often be the male partner. Again, this can antagonize supporters of Roe v. Wade. It does not, however, stop the reality of people's feelings. Another counselor recalled clients who wanted to enlist their help in memorializing "murdered babies," perhaps an alienating concept for most progressive mental health providers. While moderate and left-leaning people may find these beliefs odd, untenable, or even absurd, reasonable people hold them, and they come up in counseling and therapy.

(a male psychologist in Louisiana)

Regardless of whether we focus on distractions or more proximal direct causation, mental health professionals are now facing many clients whose anxiety, depression, and other symptoms are, at least in part, related to political realities. In some instances, couples and families have been fractured or pushed to the breaking point by political hatred. For some, politicized topics are ubiquitous and almost inescapable, the way that tensions in the United States were following the 9/11 attacks nearly 25 years ago. The 24-hour news cycle, social media, never-ending political campaigning, and the politicization of issues like climate change, reproductive rights, ongoing wars, and the COVID epidemic have directly impacted much of our population. The constant exposure to political stress has been associated with an "increased risk of anxiety, depression, and poor lifestyle choices" (Brietzke, 2022).

Often, clinicians and counselors may overlook the sources of stress that their clients face because their own experiences and world views limit their understanding. Just as White clinicians must learn to understand the difficulties that Black clients face from racism and microaggression, clinicians may remain unfamiliar with the sources of stress that our politically diverse clients face. For example, for conservatives, getting a college education can be a culturally challenging experience. On college and university campuses, liberal students and faculty are often the majority. At many institutions in North America, growing numbers of conservative students report the campus environment as increasingly hostile and unwelcoming (Manbeck et al., 2018). Right-leaning students and faculty are more likely to experience feelings of marginalization, isolation, and open hostility on predominantly liberal college campuses. Studies have consistently indicated that liberals' stereotypes about conservatives are inaccurate and usually err in the direction of categorizing them as more extreme (Graham, Nosek, & Haidt, 2012; Scherer, Windschitl, & Graham, 2015). The phenomenon of banning speakers from appearing on campuses because of their politics or stance on social issues has taken hold on many campuses. Conservative voices are often silenced in classrooms, and right-leaning students are criticized as being oppressors, racists, and terrorists. Johnson et al. (2017) describes this as "political Manichaeism," which is the process of demonizing those with opposing political ideologies as inhuman and evil. Too often the liberal response may be, as a colleague said, "Just become progressive."

Political Stress

Politics and political discussion can become both emotionally taxing and chronically stressful (Ford et al., 2023). Political trauma may be akin to posttraumatic stress disorder (PTSD) in its symptoms and severity. However, political stress usually does not meet diagnostic criteria, nor does it qualify as an adjustment disorder where, by definition, the reaction is out of proportion to the stress.

Perhaps political stress should be conceptualized along the lines of the classic stress-diathesis model; similar, though certainly not as intense as stress from sexism or racism. Racism, for example, triggers stress through various mechanisms, significantly impacting both mental and physical health. Experiences of racism, whether through direct discrimination, microaggressions, or systemic inequalities, activate the body's stress response. This response releases stress hormones, such as cortisol, which, while helpful in acute situations, can lead to adverse health outcomes when constantly triggered by chronic exposure to racism. The persistent state of vigilance and the anticipation of racial discrimination can exacerbate this stress response, leading to a range of mental health issues, including helplessness, anxiety, depression, and symptoms akin to PTSD.

Stress, as is well known from introductory psychology classes, triggers the body's "fight or flight" response, releasing hormones like cortisol and adrenaline. While these responses are beneficial in acute situations, chronic stress can lead to dysregulation of this system, affecting brain function and mood. It can precipitate the development of mental health disorders such as anxiety and depression by altering brain chemistry, impairing the function of neurotransmitters like serotonin and dopamine. Stress can be the primary cause of some psychological problems. Stress hormones can downregulate biobehavioral functions to a degree that can induce anxiety, depression, or other disorders. Furthermore, for people with existing mental health conditions, stress can serve as a catalyst for worsening symptoms. It can reduce the effectiveness of coping mechanisms, making it more challenging to manage conditions like bipolar disorder, schizophrenia, and PTSD. Chronic stress exacerbates these conditions by reinforcing negative thought patterns, increasing susceptibility to episodes of illness, and complicating recovery.

Chronic stress can also erode social networks, diminishing perceived support and increasing isolation. Social support is vital for mental health, providing a buffer against stress. However, the behaviors associated with chronic stress, such as withdrawal, irritability, and aggression, can strain relationships, leading to a reduction in social support. Previously functional, supportive work or social relationships can fracture when political leanings are revealed and further isolate individuals. This reduction in turn exacerbates stress and its psychological impacts, creating a vicious cycle.

Furthermore, chronic stress also has a direct impact on physical health, which can further affect mental well-being. It's linked to a range of physical conditions, from heart disease to diabetes, by promoting inflammation, affecting immune function, and altering metabolic processes. These physical health issues can compound the psychological burden on an individual, creating additional sources of stress and further deteriorating mental health.

Political stress, a prevalent issue in contemporary society, has significant implications for psychological well-being. It can cause new psychological problems and exacerbate existing mental health issues through various pathways because it is ever-present. The constant bombardment of political news, especially when it's polarizing or fear-inducing, is an important contributor to chronic stress. It's increasingly difficult to disconnect from the constant media attention to political issues and viewpoints that seem intent on stoking existential fears. There's an unrelenting sense that life as we know it in our country will irrevocably change if one or the other political party is in power. The message is "Be afraid, be very afraid."

Exposure to political violence or extreme political rhetoric can induce feelings of fear, anger, or helplessness, contributing to psychological distress. Such exposure can exacerbate symptoms in individuals with pre-existing conditions like PTSD, anxiety disorders, or depression. The divisive nature of current politics can strain personal relationships, leading to a sense of isolation or loss of social support. Social support is crucial for mental health; thus, its reduction can worsen existing mental health conditions and trigger new psychological problems.

Moreover, political policies can directly impact individuals' lives, influencing factors like healthcare access, employment, and economic stability. Uncertainty or negativity surrounding these areas can increase stress, anxiety, and depressive symptoms, particularly in vulnerable populations. Neighborhoods may feel less safe or welcoming; friends and colleagues become more divided by their political views.

Additionally, the sheer volume of political content in media can lead to information overload, contributing to feelings of overwhelm and fatigue. This can lead to sleep problems, irritability, and difficulty concentrating, further impacting mental health. There would seem to be absolutely no reason to exclude this topic from the therapy space.

Politics as the Last Taboo

While therapists aim to maintain neutrality, political discussions can compromise this objective, risking the therapeutic alliance. Yet, avoiding politics can hinder therapy's effectiveness, especially when clients' concerns are intertwined with political issues. The challenge is to navigate these discussions without compromising the therapeutic environment's integrity.

Many practitioners have been interfacing with a much more politically polarized public with little or no specific training to guide them. This became apparent after the 2016 election in the United States (Farber, 2018). Yet, unfortunately, little was done to assist mental health professionals in recognizing their own biases or to provide any training or guidance regarding politically charged situations.

Even mental health professionals who don't consider themselves to have a particular political affiliation have some sense of "right and wrong" regarding many social issues that have become embedded in politics. Social justice, access to abortion, climate change, assisted suicide, gun safety, LGBTQ+ rights, immigration, and a host of other social issues that affect so many of our lives are woven into our political discourse. Increasingly, social issues are now a focus of legislation in many of our states and directly impact our clients. Because so many of us may also be impacted by these issues, the idea of a "blank slate" may be a difficult façade to maintain.

In discussions with colleagues, we've heard repeated stories from mental health professionals working with clients struggling with our contentious political environment. As Brietzke (2022) noted, "Patients began to ask about my views on COVID controversies, Donald Trump's mental health, freedom of speech, the Black Lives Matter movement, and neutral pronouns." Clients intuitively want to sense where we stand on certain issues before they decide whether or what to share about their beliefs and experiences.

One erroneous belief, to be discussed in later chapters, is that if therapists could somehow "convert" a client to the "correct way of thinking," this could immunize them from political turmoil. Apart from the ethics and practicality issues, mental disorders and life problems aren't limited to either side of the political spectrum. Adherence to a political philosophy does not immunize anyone from depression, anxiety, relationship challenges, trauma, grief, and all the other experiences that bring people to seek professional help. Some research suggests higher rates of mental health disorders, such as anxiety and depression, in people who identify as liberals (Kirkegaard, 2022; Bernardi, 2021; Schlenker, Chambers, & Lee, 2012), and there is a higher likelihood that liberals will seek counseling or psychotherapy. There's speculation about this correlation and how to account for those findings (Briki & Dagot, 2022). Still, liberals are certainly more likely to find a therapist who has a similar world view. As we noted in the previous chapter, mental health providers are primarily liberal, and this shared perspective makes a stronger bond between a therapist and client, which often leads to a better outcome in therapy.

Solomonov and Barber (2019) concluded that: "Politics play an important role in therapeutic processes as in-session political discussions are common and perceived political similarity may affect decisions to self-disclose and alliance quality" (p. 1508). Their study found that most therapists (87%) discussed political issues in-session with clients, and 63% disclosed their political orientation either explicitly (21%) or implicitly (42%). Those therapists who shared their political leanings reported a stronger alliance with like-minded clients (Soloman & Barber, 2019, pp. 1515–1516). These findings suggest that political discourse is an important aspect of working with many of our clients and that training and supervision are necessary to help us ethically and effectively incorporate this skill into our work. Rather than avoiding this topic, we believe it needs to become part of our approach to better understand, connect with, and assist our clients. It's also clear that many mental health professionals have been deeply affected personally by current political divisions, policy decisions, and animosity and could benefit from supportive guidance and supervision in how to effectively self-disclose in the therapeutic space.

How Not to Respond to a Client with Different Values than Yours

SHEILA: A CASE STUDY

In 2021 when COVID vaccines became widely available, I experienced a significant "melt-down" with a client with whom I'd been working for many months. Sheila was a single woman in her mid-50s who came to our in-office sessions with an oxygen tank and breathing mask for treatment of COPD. She had been on oxygen for almost a year and had several emergency hospitalizations due to breathing problems. Due to COVID, I closed my office and transferred clients to a telehealth platform to continue our work.

When the COVID vaccines became widely available, my first thought was about this client since she was already so vulnerable to respiratory problems. Of all my clients, she was the one I was most grateful would finally have some protection from the virus. I asked if she had been able to get vaccinated and was stunned when she replied, "I'm not getting a vaccine; they're putting microchips in them that track you."

My response was not my finest moment as a therapist. "Are you nuts? That's just a ridiculous conspiracy theory. How would that even work? The vaccine vials have more than one dose, so how would there be ANY way to track which one you got!?" I went on like that for several minutes until I realized Sheila had been uncharacteristically silent for some time.

I had lost it. I was shocked and angry that anyone would perpetrate such a ridiculous idea, one that could endanger people like Sheila. I was deeply concerned about the risk she was taking by avoiding the vaccine. I apologized for my rant. The damage was done, however, and our work together suffered. A few months later, she disappeared and didn't respond to my outreach calls.

(Psychologist, Florida)

Many clinicians have stories about someone they've been working with whose politicized views have presented an unexpected challenge to the therapeutic relationship. A right-leaning colleague shared his struggle to use the requested pronouns with a client who was gender non-binary and wanted to be referred to as "they/them." A liberal therapist providing telehealth therapy found herself distracted by a large Trump flag in the background of her client's home. We've been confronted with the grief and anger many people are feeling about climate change, COVID policies, equality and civil rights, free speech, gun violence, the future of democracy, and other issues that are embedded in our politics. Political divisions have become more personal for our clients, colleagues, and us.

Most mental health training programs provide little guidance on navigating the politically charged issues that are increasingly arising in the therapy space. Perhaps more than any issue, politics is our last taboo. As a result, many mental health professionals feel unprepared and uncertain how to effectively discuss political topics with clients in an ethical, therapeutic manner. Some therapists have reacted by avoiding or redirecting any talk of politics, viewing it as a diversion from the "real issues." Others have refused clients based solely on their political affiliation, raising ethical concerns about bias and discrimination. Overall, there is a lack of clear best practices for addressing this new challenge. As we've noted, however, research shows that clients frequently do discuss politics in therapy. As such, there is a growing need to develop competencies for thoughtfully and appropriately incorporating political discourse into clinical practice when relevant to the client's needs.

To best support clients in this era of polarization, the mental health field must prioritize training practitioners in how to ethically and skillfully discuss political concerns impacting emotional well-being. This includes:

- Developing competencies for creating a safe space to process charged political topics relevant to the client's presenting issues.
- Maintaining objectivity in the therapy space while allowing exploration of different perspectives.

- Helping clients cope with acute stress from dramatic political events/changes without requiring their conformity to specific ideologizes or political beliefs.
- Addressing political issues underlying specific mental health symptoms, including personality disorders, bipolar issues, depression, and suspiciousness.
- Supporting clients going through major life transitions influenced or dictated by politics or political realities.
- Avoiding attempts to change clients' political beliefs in order to work within their world view.

Unfortunately, there is no evidence that any of our mental health professions are meeting these minimal goals. The political sphere has become intertwined with many individuals' innermost values, senses of identity, and life experiences in an unprecedented way. As counselors and therapists, we can no longer avoid this critical contextual factor shaping the mental health of our clients and society. The way forward requires evolving our practices to thoughtfully and ethically integrate this dimension of human experience.

Mental health professionals must be better prepared to acknowledge and address these concerns directly as they are brought into the therapy space. Those we serve will look to us for guidance and support in coping more effectively with the impact on their well-being and relationships with others in this age of political polarization. In the following chapters, we focus on how to prepare ourselves to assist our clients.

Summary

The therapy space is a setting that facilitates open communication, emotional processing, and self-reflection, enabling clients to explore their inner worlds, confront challenges, and embark on a journey of self-discovery and healing. Political discussions can challenge the neutrality of the therapy space, possibly compromising the therapeutic alliance. The current political climate can affect mental health, introducing stress and concerns that hinder the therapeutic process. Therapists now face evolving challenges of needing to navigate political discussions carefully, while doing so without compromising the therapy space's integrity.

References

American Psychological Association. (2023). *Using psychology to understand and fight health misinformation: An APA consensus statement.* www.apa.org/pubs/reports/health-misinformation

Bernardi, L. (2021). Depression and political predispositions: Almost blue? *Party Politics, 27*(6), 1132–1143.

Birbilis, J. M. (2018). When psychology and politics commingle. *Journal of Clinical Psychology, 74*(5), 730–733. https://doi.org/10.1002/jclp.22602

Brietzke, E. (2022, March 8). *Political polarization is affecting mental health.* Queen's University, Queen's Gazette.

Briki, W., & Dagot, L. (2022). Conservatives are happier than liberals: The mediating role of perceived goal progress and flow experience – A pilot study. *Current Psychology, 41*(3), 1267. https://doi.org/10.1007/s12144-020-00652-0

Chamberlain, L. (2021). *Practicing psychotherapy: Lessons on helping patients and growing as a professional.* New York, NY: Routledge.

Cuijpers, P., Reijnders, M., & Huibers, M. J. H. (2019). The role of common factors in psychotherapy outcomes. *Annual Review of Clinical Psychology, 15*(1), 207–231. https://doi.org/10.1146/annurev-clinpsy-050718-095424

Farber, B. A. (2018). 'Clowns to the left of me, jokers to the right': Politics and psychotherapy, 2018. *Journal of Clinical Psychology, 74*(5), 714–721. https://doi.org/10.1002/jclp.22600

Ford, B. Q., Feinberg, M., Lassetter, B., Thai, S., & Gatchpazian, A. (2023, January 23). The political is personal: The costs of daily politics. Journal of Personality and Social Psychology: Attitudes and Social Cognition, https://doi.org/10.1037/pspa0000335

Gabriel, T. (2023, October 7). Two families got fed up with their states' politics. So they moved out. *NYTimes.com.* www.nytimes.com/2023/10/07/us/politics/politics-states-moving.html?

Graham, J., Nosek, B., & Haidt, J. (2012). The moral stereotypes of liberals and conservatives: Exaggeration of differences across the political spectrum. *PLoS One, 7*(12). https://doi.org/10.1371/journal.pone.0050092

Johnson, K. M., Moryl, M., Ebersole, C. R., Haidt, J., Iyer, R., & Graham, J. (2017). *Measuring political prejudice: Political Manichaeism predicts ideological hostility toward conservatives and liberals.* Unpublished manuscript. University of Southern California.

Kindsvatter, A. (2024, April 30). *Fidelity to individual psychotherapy patients in a time of ideological extremism.* Foundation Against Intolerance & Racism. https://news.fairforall.org/p/fidelity-to-individual-psychotherapy

Kirkegaard, E. O. W. (2022, January 29). *The conservative advantage in mental health keeps replicating.* https://emilkirkegaard.dk/en/2022/01/the-conservative-advantage-in-mental-health-keeps-replicating/

Lee, K., Ashton, M. C., Griep, Y., & Edmonds, M. (2018). Personality, religion, and politics: An investigation in 33 countries. *European Journal of Personality, 32*(2), 100–115. https://doi.org/10.1002/per.2142

Manbeck, K. E., Kanter, J. W., Kuczynski, A. M., Fine, L., Corey, M. D., & Maitland, D. W. M. (2018). Improving relations among conservatives and liberals on a college campus: A preliminary trial of a contextual-behavioral intervention. *Journal of Contextual Behavioral Science, 10*, 120–125. https://doi.org/10.1016/j.jcbs.2018.10.106

Novotney, A. (2023, October). 'The young people feel it in their bones': A look at the mental health impact of anti-trans legislation. *Monitor on Psychology, 54*(7), 26–2.

Panagopoulos, C., & Weinschenk, A. C. (2023). Health and election outcomes: Evidence from the 2020 U.S. Presidential Election [Article]. *Political Research Quarterly*, *76*(2), 712–724. https://doi.org/10.1177/10659129221113256

Scherer, A. M., Windschitl, P. D., & Graham, J. (2015). An ideological house of mirrors: Political stereotypes as exaggerations of motivated social cognition differences. *Social Psychological and Personality Science*, *6*(2), 201–209. https://doi.org/10.1177;1948550614549385

Schlenker, B. R., Chambers, J. R., & Le, B. M. (2012). Conservatives are happier than liberals, but why? Political ideology, personality, and life satisfaction. *Journal of Research in Personality*, 46(2), 127–146.

Smith, K. B. (2022). Politics is making us sick: The negative impact of political engagement on public health during the Trump administration. *PLoS One*, *17*(1), e0262022. https://doi.org/10.1371/journal.pone.0262022

Solomonov, N., & Barber, J. P. (2019). Conducting psychotherapy in the Trump era: Therapists' perspectives on political self-disclosure, the therapeutic alliance, and politics in the therapy room. *Journal of Clinical Psychology*, *75*, 1508–1518. https://doi.org/10.1002/jclp.22801

6

EMPATHY IN COUNSELING THE POLITICIZED CLIENT

Affective Polarization and the Partisan Client

As the previous chapters have argued, working with politically partisan mental health clients presents unique challenges for therapists and counselors. Unfortunately, these problems are likely to become more common in the future. *Affective polarization* appears to be increasing in many places across the world (Garzia, Ferreira da Silva, & Maye, 2023). Affective polarization refers to the phenomenon where people develop strong negative feelings and hostility toward those with opposing political views beyond mere disagreement on issues (Mason, 2013). Affective polarization is characterized by emotional reactions, social distancing, stereotyping, and too often, a dehumanization of those who are different from ourselves (Martherus, Martinez, Piff, & Theodoridis, 2021).

How do we best treat highly affectively politicized clients? There is at this point very little in the way of "best practices" to guide the mental health practitioner. As we did in a much earlier volume (McCown & Chamberlain, 2000) we believe that when there are no clear professional guidelines regarding what works, a good place to start is to ask experienced practitioners. The present effort involves discussions with counselors and therapists who have been open about their strategies, successes, and failures with clients who may hold strong political beliefs. The account is qualitative because there is insufficient data and guidelines to suggest an evidence-based approach. There are no firmly established guidelines for navigating the often-tricky path that we tread when politically rancorous clients have pressing mental health needs. Yet many of the strategies that successful professionals employ will already be familiar to counselors and therapists. They are not magical, but they do nothing if they are

DOI: 10.4324/9781032651217-6

untried. Their power is "merely" that they may work for many partisan clients as effectively as they work for others.

We have divided our discussion regarding counseling highly political, affectively polarized clients into various topics over the following five chapters. This chapter focuses on what works for moderately polarized clients, meaning that they are what we label "Stage One" or "Stage Two" in the affective polarization process. These are clients who identify, often strongly, with a political viewpoint that is becoming a central focus in their lives. They show some degree of affective polarization that may occur outside of the political process, an important distinction (Rudolph & Hetherington, 2021). For example, these clients typically prefer to associate primarily with people like themselves on social media. They may have started to feel angry toward those who are different from themselves and hold different views. While they may be only mildly toxic to those around them, this toxicity can build up and become more disruptive. What differentiates them from more severely partisan clients is that they still have some degree of respect for others who are different. They show few or no traces of dehumanizing their opponents. They also can question their political leaders and fellow adherents.

The goal of therapy with clients who have this level of emotional partisanship is the same as with almost all clients, regardless of their political beliefs. Foremost, we want to treat their presenting problems. The therapist does not try to implicitly change these people's political beliefs. There is no agenda except assisting the client in managing their difficulties, whatever they may be. Interventions from the therapist that speak directly about the effect of these clients' political leanings would be guided by specific problems raised by the client. For example politics becomes an appropriate topic for counseling when a client notices that there are tensions with a family member because of political differences.

Usually, though not always, clients at this depth of partisanship are able to gain an additional benefit from their work in the therapy space. During therapy, they can often achieve a deeper capacity to empathize with people whom they oppose. They can begin to recognize the complexity associated with diverse opinions. They can also begin to challenge their own thoughts and extreme behaviors. They become, as one therapist noted, "simply more reasonable people, just better people all around." While this additional benefit is never a specific goal of therapy or the criteria of therapeutic success, it can occur frequently and is an added benefit.

When clients are even more affectively polarized on this underlying spectrum of political involvement, they may need a more extensive form of treatment approaches. These more extreme clients have a lower likelihood of developing empathic responses for people who are different from themselves. They are frequently unquestioning adherents to an ideology, activist group, and/or charismatic leader. By this time in their progression, their adherence to an overriding group is usually unquestionable, and their disdain for others who are not like themselves is toxic. They represent the end of the process where they have embraced extreme ideology or have based their identity more on their political affiliations. We have labeled these people as *highly toxic partisans* and note that they typically need a more in-depth level of intervention, described in the following chapters, including depolarization training discussed in Chapter 10. Therapy for these people is often based on helping them find different social systems where they can feel empowered and meet their needs. It also involves steps to contain their toxic behavior toward people around them. Specific problems, including partisanship in the family, dating and politics, and the partisan client with psychiatric diagnoses, are further discussed in later chapters.

Goals for the Politicized Client

Counselors and therapists who have worked with people who they consider politically partisan often note that it seems almost natural to want to change their clients' beliefs. This is a response that often occurs because, as one counselor stated, "Fringe beliefs just stick out like a sore thumb. You are drawn to do something because these beliefs are simply so crazy."

Yet experienced counselors and therapists who have successfully worked with highly politicized clients are all but uniform in their belief that this mindset will not work. *The goals for therapy with highly partisan people, as with any person, should be to treat clients' presenting problems.* This may not always be possible when the client is highly affectively polarized, yet it remains a goal.

The core of therapeutic work with partisan people lies in addressing the client's presenting problems and symptoms, while attempting to ensure that their political ideologies do not cloud the clinician's judgment or interfere with the treatment process. The focus is essential for establishing a solid therapeutic alliance where the client feels understood, respected, and valued, not judged or dismissed for their political beliefs. Such an approach facilitates a safe environment where people feel comfortable and safe sharing their thoughts and feelings, which is crucial for effective therapy (Chamberlain, 2021).

When engaging with clients holding partisan views, counselors and therapists must employ a keen sense of self-awareness and reflexivity. This stance requires recognizing and setting aside personal biases and preconceptions to remain fully present and empathetic to the client's experience. This is not to say that counselors must agree with or endorse the client's political stance. Instead, they should strive to understand the role these beliefs play in the client's life and how this affects their thoughts, feelings, and decisions. By focusing on the client's emotional and psychological needs, mental health professionals can navigate the therapeutic process without allowing political differences to impede progress.

> It has to be about treating the person, not their politics. You respect the system and values they have, only intruding on their worldviews when there are no other options. And you have to do this with some beliefs you might find creepy.
> *(A Social Worker in the South)*

Therapists recognize that political beliefs often hold deep personal significance for people, always intertwined with their identity, values, and experiences (Westwood & Peterson, 2022). These beliefs influence clients' worldviews, relationships, and, indeed, their mental health. However, the goal of therapy is usually not to challenge or change these views but to help the client understand how they relate to the client's presenting issues. By maintaining a nonjudgmental stance, therapists can explore how political beliefs impact the client's life without minimizing or disregarding their importance. This approach respects clients' autonomy and the realities of their lives.

Yet, it is also reasonable to hope that clients themselves gain an increased sense of empathy and a more flexible understanding of the world. Empathy is a critical component of psychological well-being (Martin & Johnson, 2024). It is often constricted in those with extreme viewpoints, especially toward those who are different. Partisan clients may struggle to relate to or understand the emotions and perspectives of others, particularly those outside their ideological echo chambers (Reyna, Vazquez, Vazquez, Eadeh, & Harris, 2024). Therapy aims to gently challenge this insularity, encouraging clients to step into the shoes of others to understand different life experiences and viewpoints without immediate judgment or rejection. This process is not about diluting clients' beliefs or denying their experiences but expanding their capacity for compassion and understanding, which can lead to more fulfilling interpersonal relationships and a more balanced view of the world.

Developing a more complex view of the world is a secondary therapeutic goal that is never at odds with assisting the client with their presenting problems. People with excessively partisan beliefs often see issues in black and white, lacking appreciation for different views of the nature of social, political, and personal realities (Axelrod, Daymude, & Forrest, 2021). The therapy space can provide the safety to explore these complexities, question binary thinking, and consider the multitude of factors that shape opinions, behaviors, and societal structures. This exploration can foster a more flexible mindset, enabling clients to engage more constructively with the world in the realm of therapy, particularly with clients who harbor extreme political views.

By fostering empathy and a more complex understanding of the world, therapy can play a crucial role in helping these individuals lead more balanced and harmonious lives. This not only benefits the clients themselves but also contributes to a more empathetic and understanding society, where dialogue and compassion bridge the divides of political extremism. The therapist's role is to guide this journey by creating a therapeutic environment where clients are supported and respected. By doing so, the therapist helps the client to build bridges of understanding and cultivate a more inclusive and empathetic worldview, which is essential for personal growth and for social harmony.

"Care, But Not Dismissively": Helping the Political Partisan

Counselors and clinicians of many professional identities indicate that they use a variety of therapy techniques with highly partisan people. Techniques like Socratic questioning, cognitive restructuring, and examining counterevidence can help clients identify cognitive distortions and move toward more nuanced, balanced perspectives. Mindfulness exercises that reduce emotional reactivity can also be beneficial, as can stress reduction techniques. In fact, methods and procedures do not appear to be any different from those in "ordinary" therapy. This is not surprising since the aim is not to change political views per se, but to cultivate open-mindedness, compassion, intellectual humility, and recognition that few issues are ever truly black-and-white.

Few therapeutic techniques will work without an environment of openness, empathy, and nonjudgment. Clients with firmly held political views may feel defensive if they sense the therapist is judgmental or trying to change their beliefs. The therapist should validate and honor the client's right to their own perspectives and thought processes. Active listening, reflecting back what the client expresses, and seeking to understand their beliefs and motivations can help build rapport and trust, as it does with other clients. The goal is not to argue or debate political topics, but to understand the client as a whole person. *It is never to change a client's political views.*

Mental health professionals who have successfully worked with clients with strong political opinions stress the importance of maintaining empathy. Yet they also discuss the instinctual desire for counselors and therapists to react emotionally to their client's political views. A politically progressive psychologist practicing in a rural, highly conservative area noted: "*These clients, just like all clients, respond to a therapist who cares. They blossom. But it is tough when their whole worldviews are simply wrong. Somehow, I've learned a new skill that lets me care, but not dismissively.*"

Similarly, a conservative counselor with a military background who has worked with more politically progressive clients noted:

I've worked with people whose views I don't respect. They often do things I don't understand. However, what I've seen is that by having real empathy, you can make progress regardless of what a person's politics (are). You don't dismiss their views, and you don't argue with them. You try to show you care even if you don't understand their politics.

Dismissing or invalidating a client's political beliefs may be perceived as an attack on their identity and values, potentially hindering the therapeutic relationship and progress. (NO PARAGRAPH BREAK HERE)
Unfortunately, for too many of us, it is our implicit therapy goal with clients with whom we disagree. As Chapter 3 discussed, it is human nature to want people to be "like us" and to hold our values and political views. This is because we believe our values are the most logical, just, sensible, and correct. Otherwise, we would not hold them. Consequently, even the most empathetic therapists may bristle when they work with clients who hold beliefs that substantially differ from their own.

By acknowledging that political choices are often complexly woven into a person's sense of self, counselors and therapists can foster an environment of understanding, respect, and open dialogue. This approach allows clients to explore the complexities of their political identities, the underlying motivations, and how these choices affect their overall well-being and relationships. Yet, this will not occur when we attempt to manipulate or even influence our client's politics. Our instinctive desire to make clients "more like us" as a part of a therapy outcome may be well-intentioned. This is especially true when the counselor or therapist believes that the client's views represent a social risk. However, experienced mental health professionals believe it is impractical and counterproductive.

As also noted by so many mental health professionals, an overall strategy that effective therapists seem to use with partisan clients is to avoid confrontation or direct arguing. This is usually unproductive with clients (Goldman, Vaz, & Rousmaniere, 2021; Mösler, Poppek, Leonhard, & Collet, 2023; Newman, 2013). Instead, many effective practitioners typically strive to allow the client to experience an empathic relationship free of political demands and criticism. As with other clients, curiosity and empathic listening creates the therapeutic space for personal growth in our clients. A right-leaning counselor noted regarding her liberal clients:

Part of me feels if they just didn't have these screwball beliefs, they would usually be fine. But I've learned it doesn't help to preach. I can't just tell them to go to church, and all will be great, like some Christian counselors do. What helps is to listen with an open heart and try to see the world from their eyes.

Empathy, regardless of the counselor's own beliefs, has many functions that combat partisan biases. An empathic stance works regardless of the specific orientation of the practitioner or the details of her clinical theories. Somewhat oddly, many therapists still associate empathy primarily with client-centered approaches to therapy. Since their orientation to treatment may be toward another set of theories, they may feel that the concept of empathy is not especially important for their work (Chen & Giblin, 2018). This is a narrow view. Empathetic listening, defined not merely as a passive act but as an active engagement, forms the bedrock of most successful therapeutic relationships, regardless of the technique and theoretical orientation of the practitioner (Clark, 2023).

A counselor in the upper Midwest United States stated how applying empathy with clients changed her practice:

I used to try, maybe not so consciously, to change the beliefs of my clients. I'm a liberal through and through. I thought, 'How the hell do these people believe the crap that they do?' But honestly, no one ever changed when I did that. What works for me is showing respect and caring. That's when people started to make real changes.

Empathy is essential because it involves a demonstration of genuine respect (Elliott, Bohart, Larson, Muntigl, & Smoliak, 2023). This respect may be something that has been lacking in the lives of highly partisan people. A foundational goal of therapy is to encourage clients to show this respect toward others in their social worlds. Counselors and therapists also need to respect their clients' values if they are to show empathy. This does not mean that they must endorse these values or find them reasonable. Nor should they pretend to endorse them or gently smile when clients' beliefs are seemingly irrational or absurd. Instead, mental health professionals need to respect the role of individual choices in political decisions and ideology. For many people, their political beliefs and affiliations are not merely superficial preferences but rather a reflection of their core values, worldviews, and life experiences. Counselors and therapists must respect the process that led to their development and also respect the individual's choices. Political choices often stem from an individual's upbringing, cultural background, personal values, personality, and deeply held belief systems. As indicated in Chapter 2, even genetics may be part of this equation. These factors shape how a person perceives and interprets the world around them, influencing their stance on various social, economic, and environmental issues. Political choices can become an integral part of an individual's identity, representing their ideals, aspirations, and the causes they feel enthusiastic about.

Counselors and therapists whose goal is that their clients will change their political sentiments are not pursuing a goal congruent with genuine respect and empathy. They often fail to provide the experience of empathy in the therapy space, disallowing politicized clients the freedom to examine their feelings, biases, and other issues. The uniqueness of the therapy space is that it allows an entirely novel experience for most people. Often, for the first time, clients given this respect can express their thoughts and feelings without either having to defend themselves or feeling pressure from others to endorse specific views. In the therapy space, clients can become empowered to develop their values independent of social echo chambers or peer group expectations. Since confrontation and defensiveness may encourage clients to entrench more firmly, the aim is to avoid conflict and promote self-reflection.

As a very liberal client noted after several months of counseling with a conservative therapist:

> What I appreciate about (my counselor) is that she let me be open about my commitment to social justice. I don't think she understands it, but she didn't attack me. I didn't have to hide my feelings because she disagreed. I think this openness helped me be more accepting of people I used to think were ignorant.

Genuine empathy is crucial because it is agnostic about the causes of political divisions. Therapists should realize that for some clients, their political choices may be closely tied to their experiences of marginalization, oppression, or privilege. Those who have faced systemic discrimination or inequalities may align themselves with political movements or parties that advocate for social justice, equal rights, and the dismantling of oppressive structures.

Conversely, people who have benefited from certain privileges may gravitate toward political ideologies that aim to maintain the status quo or protect their interests. Rarely are these choices conscious. Rather, these beliefs are embedded in their social networks, places of employment, religious beliefs, personal experiences, family histories, and other influences.

People who have lost faith in aspects of the dominant culture may cling to politics to seek a return to conditions that they once believed were more favorable. Many people feel that "their kind" is not allowed to play on a fair playing field, which can influence political feelings on both the Left and Right. Beyond this, people may have individual differences that encourage but do not mandate the development of specific political views. These may include an orientation toward the past, levels of conscientiousness, or an openness to new experiences, as previously discussed. The successful counselor is aware that political affiliations often provide their clients with a sense of belonging and connection to a broader community or group. People may derive a sense of camaraderie and solidarity from sharing similar political ideologies with others, fostering a collective identity and shared purpose. Even virtual communities in social media can help provide this identity. A sense of belonging can be essential for people seeking validation and meaning, as well as friends. Yet, this is a point that many mental health professionals do not seem to understand. Directly refuting these values is usually not helpful to the person holding them. It can deprive them of community and social support, sometimes with catastrophic results.

A very politically active social worker in a Northeast state expressed this from her experience, which is quite different from most of the clients she works with.

> I am lesbian. My partner is a woman of color. I have trans people in my family. I've had more than my share of clients who say offensive things to people in my community, and frankly, it is upsetting. I used to try to get them to change their values. The few times I managed to get them to change, you know, just a bit, you … become more mainstream. I don't think it helped them. They moved more to the center but lost friends, church, whatever. I don't think we help anyone when we deprive them of a community. Change has to be more organic.

Ultimately, embracing political choices as a facet of human identity allows change to be more organic. It promotes a more holistic and client-centered approach to mental health counseling, enabling individuals to express and integrate all aspects of their lived experiences fully. The necessity of listening and empathy, especially with clients holding extreme or partisan political views, cannot be overstated. Empathy, not debating engagement, may be the *sine qua non* of therapy with partisan clients. Therapists must cultivate a genuine listening approach that transcends mere acknowledgment of the client's words, striving instead for a deep understanding of their experiences and perspectives. Empathetic listening needs to be a consistent stance, irrespective of the therapist's personal views. It allows clients to feel genuinely heard and valued, fostering trust and openness.

For almost every client, empathy is important to the therapeutic process (Gardner, 2024). Yet this is even more essential for people who do not expect that counselors and therapists can understand them. The concept that a person can have a conversation in the therapy space where they are not judged or forced to endorse or evaluate a political opinion can sometimes be highly revealing for partisan clients. It is also mutually rewarding for counselors and therapists. As an Evangelical Christian therapist from a conservative part of the United States noted:

> When I started listening to what my liberal clients were saying, they were less defensive. Include me as well in that. I was also part of the problem. When I started listening, I became less defensive as well. I actually realized I could help people I disagreed with.

Demonstrating empathy for those who are not like us, and who may espouse ideas we find challenging or offensive, is often extremely difficult (Cabaniss, Cherry, Douglas, & Schwartz, 2011; Hill, 2014). However, the approach we advocate goes beyond simply lending a pleasant ear or sympathizing with clients. A counselor is not a friend, but a skilled practitioner engaged in a highly disciplined yet quite authentic and spontaneous procedure. Many popular accounts and therapeutic techniques differentiate between listening to understand compared to listening to form a response. What distinguishes competent mental health providers is that they can listen to understand and not merely listen. Clients can model this and learn to modify defensive responses that others outside of their tribe often consider off putting and toxic. This type of empathy involves an authentic engagement with a client's emotional world that can be difficult to manage for a highly partisan client. This can be particularly challenging yet essential for clients with strong political beliefs who are disrespectful, authoritarian, or provoking. Therapists and counselors must navigate these conversations with a balanced stance, ensuring they neither invalidate nor overly align with the client's views. A delicate balance is crucial in maintaining therapeutic alliances and effectiveness.

Empathic Neutrality and Partisan Clients

Meta-analysis suggests that empathy, measured broadly, has a moderate statistical effect on measures of client outcomes (Elliott, Bohart, Watson, & Murphy, 2018). This is a consistent finding in literature dating at least to the 1960s (Martin & Johnson, 2024). While we believe the statistical effects are probably more impressive than were found in previous meta-analyses, what is important about empathy is that it is a therapy variable that counselors and therapists can attempt to control. Withholding empathic responses may often guarantee therapeutic failure.

However, no one seems to know how to develop empathy for people whose politics are often patently offensive to us or when clients hold values that we disdain or even find repulsive. In our experience therapists who work with mildly or moderately partisan clients seem most effective when they maintain a stance of openness yet simultaneous relative emotional neutrality. Listening to clients objectively, as far as possible, without judging is often the most powerful tool a therapist or counselor has (Nienhuis et al., 2018). It is also one of the most challenging tasks a counselor can attempt to tackle when working with someone who has political views that seem onerous or irrational.

A physician who works with substance abusers and their families who have a variety of political orientations noted this difficulty:

What works for me is empathy, sure. But it has to go beyond my approach to most patients. I have to remain empathetic yet also monitor how I am feeling, what I am thinking … What is so exhausting working with (highly political) patients are the simultaneous attention you have to pay to staying neutral and not imposing your values. You have to do that, but you also have to show that you genuinely care. It is tough work and not some easy skill to master when people are saying infuriating things that insult your values.

For the mental health professional, this approach may involve a different type of client orientation than a "classic" non-directive relationship. It involves cultivating a stance identified in the literature as *empathic neutrality* (Gelso & Kanninen, 2017). This term is used because it summarizes two critical attitudes: an empathetic and respectful optimism for partisan clients and, secondly, a disciplined neutrality about reaction to political topics, as far as possible. It is very similar to the stance recommended for conducting qualitative research (Ormston, Spencer, Barnard, & Snape, 2014). What may be difficult is that this stance involves two different therapy approaches. It takes the complex skillset learned in a client-centered modality, involving reflecting and emotional unity. However, it also demands the skills of objectivity, non-emotionality, and emotional restraint, often regarding subjects that may be critical to the therapist's identity. This is not an easy task at all.

Empathic neutrality enables therapists to maintain an optimistic and empathetic stance while interacting with clients who hold firm, often highly partisan, political views. This concept emphasizes the therapist's ability to provide a supportive, validating environment without aligning with or opposing the client's political beliefs. It involves recognizing the client's emotional experiences and the intensity of their convictions without judgment, thereby fostering a safe space for exploration and personal growth. Neutrality in this context does not equate to indifference or passivity; rather, it signifies a conscious effort by the therapist to refrain from imparting personal opinions or judgment despite their "gut" reactions. This neutrality, which was long recognized by more psychoanalytic colleagues (Menaker, 1990) is crucial in maintaining a therapeutic space that is free from external judgments or biases, allowing the client to explore their beliefs without fear of criticism or persuasion. The therapist's role is to facilitate self-exploration and growth, not to challenge or alter the client's political views.

The process of empathic neutrality involves maintaining an impartial and open stance while respectfully engaging with clients who hold different political viewpoints. The mental health professional assumes a stance of objective inquiry, minimizing the counter-transferential issues that arise when the therapist believes that her position is morally superior or more logical. This approach recognizes that people see the world differently and have experiences that may not seem initially the same as our own.

Politics plays a significant role in many people's lives and as we have argued earlier, in many cases will inevitably arise as a topic in therapy. The empathic neutral therapist does not avoid political topics when they occur. Nor do they act like a "political voyeur," prodding the client to reveal a worldview that the therapist may not accept or even find credible. They remain unbiased and avoid imposing their political views on the therapeutic process. Instead, they focus on the underlying emotions, beliefs, and experiences that shape the client's perspectives, using these insights to promote healing and understanding. This approach encourages clients to feel heard and respected, irrespective of their political stance, which is crucial for building therapeutic rapport and facilitating effective intervention.

Consider a scenario where a therapist is working with Alex, a client who is deeply invested in a particular political movement, which significantly affects her mental health. Alex often expresses strong, racist opinions during sessions, which are laden with political content and sarcasm. The therapist, employing empathic neutrality, listens attentively to Alex's concerns, focusing on the emotional undertones of frustration, fear, and a sense of belonging that underpin Alex's political engagement. Rather than debating the merits of Alex's politics, the therapist explores how these views relate to her life experiences, identity, and values. The therapist's optimistic and empathetic stance, coupled with a politically neutral position, helps Alex feel understood and supported, paving the way for therapeutic progress.

The core skill of empathic neutrality is the ability to discuss political differences with clients in a nonjudgmental way without avoiding or dismissing them. Counselors should create a safe and nonjudgmental space where clients feel comfortable expressing their political beliefs and perspectives without fear of being criticized or persuaded to change their opinions. While many practitioners strive for this, they often overlook this attitude when faced with an affectively partisan client. Yet perhaps the best attitude that can be conveyed is "I don't necessarily feel the way you do. However, I will listen to you and not deride you." The message we share with the client is "I want to understand what you believe and how you came to believe it."

Empathic neutrality requires counselors to listen actively and with empathy (Gelso & Kanninen, 2017). However, they must do so regardless of whether they agree or disagree with the client's political leanings. Empathic neutrality involves suspending personal biases and refraining from imposing one's own political views on the client. Instead, counselors should strive to understand the client's perspective, motivations, and the underlying factors that shape their political beliefs.

When the client asks about the therapist's politics, the therapist should be genuine and honest. However, they should also point out that the purpose of counseling is not to help the therapist, it is to help the client better understand their problems. This is similar to the style of more psychodynamic therapists who eschew questions about personal matters. But if the client wishes to discuss this further, the therapist is non-defensive and nonjudgmental.

An example is from a psychologist in Florida. When asked about his political leanings by clients, he typically responds with

> I grew up in a conservative family and appreciate those values, but I've become more liberal leaning in my life. What I find important is to respect and accept that while we may have differences, both of us want to lead a good life for ourselves and our families.

A counselor in Texas who works with clients who have political beliefs that are divergent from hers noted this:

> Many of my clients are hardcore Republicans. We probably disagree on 100% of things. I don't advertise (what I believe), just like I don't talk about religion. If it comes up, I address it honestly. But I always try to return the focus to the client. Honestly, some of their attitudes, like about global warming and guns, I believe are really dangerous. But it doesn't help them unless I work with their presenting problems.

Importantly practitioners who advocate empathic neutrality acknowledge that individuals have the freedom to make their own political choices. Therapy should not aim to convince clients to alter their political opinions (Chamberlain, 2021). Instead, the focus should be on exploring how these beliefs impact the client's overall well-being, relationships, and functioning . This is not a decision that the counselor can make for the client. The client must determine how their views affect their life and make reasonable choices about what they believe would be helpful for them.

By adopting a stance of empathic neutrality, counselors can create an environment where clients feel respected and heard, even when discussing sensitive or controversial political topics. This approach fosters trust and open communication, enabling clients to explore the complex interplay between their political beliefs and personal experiences without fear of judgment or rejection.

A practitioner attempting empathic neutrality recognizes that partisan beliefs are partly based on their functionality for the client. They serve a role, whether that's social acceptance, completion of the self, an ability to differentiate self from others or numerous other possibilities. These beliefs also get a great deal of feedback from the person's community, reiterating the self-image of the person who holds them. This feedback, even if it is slightly negative, is often perceived by the partisan client as rewarding. The therapist or counselor realizes that he must remain as neutral as possible to these political beliefs.

The therapy space is a unique place for clients, a sanctuary of sorts, a place where they should feel safe and understood, free from judgment or bias. When therapists allow their own emotions, especially those triggered by political disagreements, to infiltrate the session, it compromises this safe space. A positive, respectful atmosphere that also emphasizes emotional neutrality helps in maintaining a nonjudgmental stance, ensuring that the therapist remains an unwavering pillar of support, irrespective of the client's political affiliations. This is essential for building therapeutic rapport and trust, cornerstones of effective therapy.

Empathic neutrality is also vital because therapists' emotional reactions to political views can easily cloud their clinical judgment. As illustrated in Chapter 2, therapists often have robust responses to clients' partisan beliefs and statements. Yet strong emotions can lead to cognitive biases, potentially skewing therapists' interpretations of clients' issues and the therapeutic interventions they choose. Caring, nonjudgmental emotional detachment allows therapists to maintain objectivity, ensuring that their therapeutic interventions are guided by clinical expertise and, if available, evidence-based practices rather than personal beliefs or emotional responses (Hill, 2014). This objectivity is crucial for the effectiveness of therapy and for the clients' overall well-being.

A counselor's ability to reduce the complex skein of emotional responses to political topics is vital for modeling effective emotional regulation. Many clients may struggle with managing emotions related to their political views, which can exacerbate their mental health issues. By demonstrating how to engage with potentially triggering content without becoming emotionally overwhelmed, therapists can provide a powerful example for clients. The positive yet neutral atmosphere of the therapy space allows an individual to be accepted without referring to politics or pushing people outside of their comfort range. The importance of reducing emotions in counseling clients who hold strong political views cannot be overstated. It ensures the maintenance of a safe and supportive therapeutic environment which helps to preserve clinical objectivity. It provides a model for effective emotional regulation. These elements are indispensable in guiding clients toward mental resilience and autonomy, highlighting the critical role of emotional neutrality in the therapeutic process.

We also recognize that we all have limits, and that part of our responsibility is knowing when we aren't able to maintain empathic neutrality with a particular client. A counselor in Colorado described working with a court-ordered client who was so agitated, angry, and confrontive that his yelling attracted attention from other professionals in the office suite she shared. When the client refused repeated requests to step outside her office and take time to calm down, she stepped out and consulted with a colleague who overheard the client's outburst and was concerned about her welfare.

I was much too shaken to be of any use to this man. I could understand his concerns, but needed to feel safe working with him and I couldn't do it.

My colleague opened the door to my office and asked him to leave or he would call building security to escort him out. Fortunately, the client left and I contacted the judge who referred the case to me and let her know that I needed to withdraw.

If we are threatened or overwhelmed by threats of violent behavior, including verbal abuse, our first concern is both our safety and that of the client. Not only does the client need our respect, but therapists also need to feel safe and respected. These situations are rare, but they do occur.

Practitioners committed to empathic neutrality recognize that political differences are a natural part of the human experience and should not be avoided or suppressed in the therapeutic setting. By embracing this approach, counselors can navigate political conversations with clients in a constructive and empathetic manner, promoting personal growth and understanding while respecting individual autonomy and diversity of thought.

A Case Example: Counseling the Anti-Vaxxer

Trey is a counselor who works in an agency that provides services for families with a member who has autism. He is working with Tiffany, a divorced mother of a 16-year-old son with moderate autism. Tiffany's presenting problems relate to her depression following her divorce and the stress that raising a son with autism has caused her. Tiffany believes that her son's autism was caused by the vaccines he received. Therefore, she has continually refused to allow her two younger children to be vaccinated. She convinced various family members regarding her beliefs in vaccines and the advantages of natural immunity. However, her unvaccinated aunt passed away from Covid-19 and her mother twice became severely ill. Despite this, Tiffany has become even more resolute in her belief that vaccines are dangerous. She is angry, demanding, and dismissive of anyone who "supports poisoning our babies."

In the initial sessions, Trey focuses on building rapport with the client, ensuring she feels understood and respected. He practiced active listening, reflecting her feelings and summarizing her statements to show that he is fully engaged and values her perspective. This approach helps establish trust and demonstrates that he is not there to judge or change her but to support her in her journey of exploration.

Once a therapeutic alliance is established, Trey gently encourages Tiffany to articulate her beliefs about vaccines, asking open-ended questions to understand the depth and source of her convictions. "What are your main concerns about vaccines?" or "Can you share how you came to believe this about vaccines?" are examples of questions that prompt self-exploration without challenging her beliefs directly.

Throughout their conversations, he makes it a point to validate Tiffany's emotions, acknowledging that her fears and concerns are real to her, regardless of the underlying facts. "It sounds like you're really worried about the safety of vaccines, and it's understandable to want to protect your health and the health of your children," he might say, emphasizing empathy and understanding.

As Tiffany becomes more comfortable, he introduces gentle Socratic questioning to encourage critical thinking. For example, he might ask, "What would evidence look like that would make you feel more comfortable with vaccines?" or "Is there a source of information you would trust to explore this further?" These questions are designed to stimulate her own cognitive processes, encouraging her to consider the validity and sources of her information.

When Tiffany expresses doubts or inconsistencies in her beliefs, he uses this opportunity to explore cognitive dissonance. For instance, if she mentions trusting her doctor for other medical issues but not for vaccines, he'd explore this discrepancy with her, asking how she reconciles these contrasting beliefs, always from a place of curiosity and not judgment. If Tiffany showed openness, he might introduce information in a very gentle, non-confrontational way. This could be as subtle as discussing the history of vaccines and their role in eradicating diseases or sharing stories of individuals who have benefited from vaccines, always ensuring the information is presented in a way that respects her autonomy and decision-making process.

Over time, through this empathic yet restrained approach, Tiffany begins to express doubts about her previous beliefs. She acknowledges the complexities of the issue and recognizes that possible misinformation might have influenced her fear. She also discussed her feelings about whether her aunt, who passed away, might have avoided a vaccination because of the aunt's political beliefs. Encouraged by the safe space she and Trey have created, she takes steps to independently research credible sources, eventually arriving at a more balanced and informed perspective aligned with mainstream medical recommendations.

By the end of the sessions, Tiffany's viewpoint on vaccines had shifted significantly. She has not been coerced or criticized into changing her beliefs. Trey never contradicted anything she said. Yet she has embarked on a self-guided journey of questioning and learning facilitated by an environment of empathy and understanding. This transformation is more likely to be sustainable and empowering, as it stems from her critical thinking and agency. She also allowed her children to be vaccinated, a decision she made by herself without prompting from her counselor or anyone else.

Summary

Working with politically partisan clients presents unique challenges for mental health professionals, particularly as affective polarization increases in society.

The chapter emphasizes that the primary goal when working with these clients must remain treating their presenting problems, not changing their political beliefs. Success in therapy with partisan clients requires counselors and therapists to maintain a careful balance: they must demonstrate genuine empathy and create a safe, nonjudgmental environment while avoiding any attempt to influence or challenge their clients' political views, even when those views conflict with their own values.

The concept of "empathic neutrality" emerges as a crucial therapeutic stance when working with politically partisan clients. This approach combines empathetic and respectful optimism with disciplined neutrality regarding political topics. It requires therapists to suspend their personal biases and emotional reactions while maintaining authentic engagement with clients' experiences. The chapter illustrates that this dual approach—being both emotionally present and politically neutral—allows clients to feel truly heard and respected, often for the first time experiencing a space where they can express their thoughts without having to defend themselves or feel pressure to endorse specific views.

Successful therapy with partisan clients recognizes that political beliefs often serve important functions in clients' lives, providing community, identity, and a sense of belonging. The chapter demonstrates through various case examples that when therapists maintain empathic neutrality and focus on treating presenting problems rather than attempting to change political views, clients often naturally develop more balanced perspectives and even greater empathy for others. This process must be organic and client-driven, as attempting to directly challenge or change clients' political beliefs can be counterproductive and potentially harmful, possibly depriving them of important support systems and community connections.

References

Axelrod, R., Daymude, J. J., & Forrest, S. (2021). Preventing extreme polarization of political attitudes. *Proceedings of the National Academy of Sciences of the United States of America, 118*(50), 1–11. https://doi.org/10.1073/pnas.2102139118

Cabaniss, D. L., Cherry, S., Douglas, C. J., & Schwartz, A. R. (2011). *Psychodynamic psychotherapy: A clinical manual*. Wiley-Blackwell.

Chamberlain, L. L. (2021). Practicing psychotherapy: Lessons on helping clients and growing as a professional. Routledge/Taylor & Francis Group. https://ulm.idm.oclc.org/login?url=https://search.ebscohost.com/login.aspx?direct=true&db=psyh&AN=2020-44155-000&site=ehost-live

Chen, M.-w., & Giblin, N. J. (2018). *Individual counseling and therapy: Skills and techniques* (3rd ed.). New York, NY: Routledge/Taylor & Francis Group.

Clark, A. J. (2023). *Empathy and mental health: An integral model for developing therapeutic skills in counseling and psychotherapy*. Routledge. https://doi.org/10.4324/9781003168355

Elliott, R., Bohart, A. C., Larson, D. G., Muntigl, P., & Smoliak, O. (2023). Empathic reflection. In C. E. Hill & J. C. Norcross (Eds.), *Psychotherapy skills and methods that work* (pp. 99–137). Oxford University Press. https://doi.org/10.1093/oso/978019 7611012.003.0005

Elliott, R., Bohart, A. C., Watson, J. C., & Murphy, D. (2018). Therapist empathy and client outcome: An updated meta-analysis. *Psychotherapy, 55*(4), 399.

Gardner, J. (2024). Forms and transformations of empathy: Subtleties and complexities of empathic communication. *Psychoanalysis, Self and Context, 19*(1), 80–93. https://doi.org/10.1080/24720038.2023.2266711

Garzia, D., Ferreira da Silva, F., & Maye, S. (2023). Affective polarization in comparative and longitudinal perspective. *Public Opinion Quarterly, 87*(1), 219–231. https://doi.org/10.1093/poq/nfad004

Gelso, C. J., & Kanninen, K. M. (2017). Neutrality revisited: On the value of being neutral within an empathic atmosphere. *Journal of Psychotherapy Integration, 27*(3), 330.

Goldman, R. N., Vaz, A., & Rousmaniere, T. (2021). Exercise 8: Empathic conjectures. In *Deliberate practice in emotion-focused therapy* (pp. 93–100). American Psychological Association. https://doi.org/10.1037/0000227-010

Hill, C. E. (2014). *Helping skills: Facilitating exploration, insight, and action* (4th ed.). American Psychological Association.

Martherus, J. L., Martinez, A. G., Piff, P. K., & Theodoridis, A. G. (2021). Party animals? Extreme partisan polarization and dehumanization. *Political Behavior, 43*(2), 517–540. https://doi.org/10.1007/s11109-019-09559-4

Martin, D. G., & Johnson, E. A. (2024). *Counseling and therapy skills*. Waveland Press.

Mason, L. (2013). The rise of uncivil agreement: Issue versus behavioral polarization in the American electorate. *American Behavioral Scientist, 57*(1), 140–159. https://doi.org/10.1177/0002764212463363

McCown, W. G., & Chamberlain, L. L. (2000). *Best possible odds: Contemporary treatment strategies for gambling disorders*. John Wiley & Sons Inc. https://ulm.idm.oclc.org/login?url=https://search.ebscohost.com/login.aspx?direct=true&db=psyh&AN=2000-07443-000&site=ehost-live

Menaker, E. (1990). Transference, countertransference, and therapeutic efficacy in relation to self-disclosure by the analyst. In G. Stricker & M. Fisher (Eds.), *Self-disclosure in the therapeutic relationship* (pp. 103–115). Plenum Press. https://doi.org/10.1007/978-1-4899-3582-3_8

Mösler, T., Poppek, S., Leonhard, C., & Collet, W. (2023). Reflective skills, empathy, wellbeing, and resilience in cognitive-behavior therapy trainees participating in mindfulness-based self-practice/self-reflection. *Psychological Reports, 126*(6), 2648–2668. https://doi.org/10.1177/00332941221094482

Newman, C. F. (2013). Core competencies in cognitive-behavioral therapy: Becoming a highly effective and competent cognitive-behavioral therapist. Routledge/Taylor & Francis Group. https://doi.org/10.4324/9780203107447

Nienhuis, J. B., Owen, J., Valentine, J. C., Winkeljohn Black, S., Halford, T. C., Parazak, S. E., Budge, S., & Hilsenroth, M. (2018). Therapeutic alliance, empathy, and genuineness in individual adult psychotherapy: A meta-analytic review. *Psychotherapy Research, 28*(4), 593–605.

Ormston, R., Spencer, L., Barnard, M., & Snape, D. (2014). The foundations of qualitative research. *Qualitative Research Practice: A Guide for Social Science Students and Researchers, 2*(7), 52–55.

Reyna, C., Vazquez, K., Vazquez, M., Eadeh, F., & Harris, K. (2024). Left and right ideological orientations as intragroup strategies of cultural preservation and promotion. *Social and Personality Psychology Compass, 18*(6). https://doi.org/10.1111/spc3.12976

Rudolph, T. J., & Hetherington, M. J. (2021). Affective polarization in political and nonpolitical settings. *International Journal of Public Opinion Research, 33*(3), 591–606. https://doi.org/10.1093/ijpor/edaa040

Westwood, S. J., & Peterson, E. (2022). The inseparability of race and partisanship in the United States. *Political Behavior, 44*(3), 1125–1147. https://doi.org/10.1007/s11109-020-09648-9

7
PARTISANSHIP AND GRIEF

The Nature of Grief

Almost everyone has experienced grief in their lives. Defining grief is often difficult because the experience is so subjective and personal, drawing on our entire history of human uniqueness (Lamia, 2022). Grief is probably best defined as a complex biopsychosocial process involving intense sorrow, yearning, and adjustment to the loss of a loved one, relationship, or cherished belief (Shear, 2012). While often associated with death, people can experience grief in response to any major loss or life transition. For example, people can grieve a job transition, a move, or even the end of a period of their lives, such as childhood or adolescence. The experience of grief is highly individual, influenced by factors like attachment style, culture, personality, and past experiences with loss (Bonanno & Kaltman, 2001).

Most bereaved people navigate grief with resilience, eventually finding healthy ways to make meaning, maintain bonds with the deceased, and move forward with living (Neimeyer, 2019). Approximately 10%, however, may experience prolonged grief disorder, marked by unrelenting yearning, trouble accepting the loss, emotional numbness, bitterness, and identity disruption more than a year later (Prigerson, Kakarala, Gang, & Maciejewski, 2021).

Lamia (2022) highlights the central role of personal identity in grieving. Losing a loved one or a core part of one's sense of self can shatter assumptions about the world. Lamia describes how, despite its subjectivity and uniqueness for each griever, grief often activates an intense search for both stability and meaning. The bereaved person tries to make sense of the loss and emptiness, eventually trying to reconstruct their identities in ways that make sense to them.

DOI: 10.4324/9781032651217-7

This process may be lifelong, in contrast to the time limited assumptions of the famous "stages-of-grief" model (Kübler-Ross, 1974), which has little empirical evidence.

In the past, many grieving people found meaning in religion, community, or spirituality. They may have wanted to memorialize the departed person through personal or social acts. They also took comfort in family, communities, and physical reminders of the past. A current option is to find meaning and relief from grief in political extremism. In this quest, some people may turn to rigid belief systems, tribalism, or scapegoating to cope with the identity that has been damaged or shattered by grief.

Grief Misused

Identifying strongly with an ideological in-group can provide belonging, meaning, and psychological safety for people struggling with loss and uncertainty (Hogg, 2014). Extremist narratives tend to frame the in-group as unfairly aggrieved and oppressed by malevolent out-groups, fostering an "us vs. them" mentality (Berger, 2018). For those grappling with intense grief, the simplicity of this good vs. evil moral framing may hold intuitive appeal.

Anger and blame toward perceived enemies can provide an outlet for painful emotions and a unifying sense of purpose (Mancini, 2019). As Lamia (2022) notes, grieving people may resort to "all-or-nothing" thinking and cling to rigid beliefs as a defense against overwhelming emotions. Fused with personal grievances, someone with cognitive rigidity can fuel ideological hatred of out-groups, heightening the potential for dehumanization and violence.

Rigid partisan beliefs may provide a sense of certainty, purpose, and control in the face of a shattered assumptive world (Janoff-Bulman, 1992), but this comes at the cost of empathy and openness to other perspectives. Entrenched polarization makes it difficult to build "communities of shared mourning" where grief and vulnerability can be processed collectively. The breakdown of shared reality and inability to communicate constructively across lines of difference compounds experiences of loss and distress.

The case study, Julia, that follows, illustrates the way that grief can be fused with political beliefs in a manner that prevents a person from finding closure following a loss.

Julia, a 38-year-old woman with a background in environmental science, lived in a suburban area of the South known for high concentrations of environmental toxins. Julia had always been moderately active in local environmental initiatives, voting for more environmentally oriented ecological transparency. She had a close and supportive relationship with her mother, a nurse, who was a significant influence in her life. Her mother shared her environmental sentiments and often acted as her best friend as they grew older.

When Julia's mother was diagnosed with an aggressive form of brain cancer and passed away within eight months, Julia was devastated. She felt she was without a rudder, a role model, and a best friend. Her intense grief and profound sense of vulnerability led her to cope by researching potential causes of her mother's cancer, strongly believing it was linked to environmental toxins that were common in her area. She was not certain why, but she became almost obsessed with this topic, sometimes reading several hours a day, taking copious notes.

Julia's grief soon channeled into an intense focus on environmental issues. She began spending significant amounts of time researching ecological toxins, pollution, and their probable links to cancer. She transformed her interest into an obsession, as she sought answers and meaning in her mother's death.

Over time, Julia's beliefs became more extreme. She began to watch YouTube videos with scientifically questionable content. She also began endorsing more radical environmental views, joining online communities that shared her concerns and often propagated conspiracy theories about government and corporate cover-ups of environmental hazards. Her homegrown activism intensified, and she became an outspoken advocate, participating in online protests and campaigns that promoted extreme measures to combat environmental problems..

Her rhetoric grew increasingly aggressive and alarmist while also losing focus. She eventually endorsed a view that vaccines had caused her mother's cancer, and she became obsessed with banning them, or at least telling people about their "dangers."

This shift in beliefs and behaviors started to alienate Julia from her former friends and social circles. Friends and family found it difficult to engage with someone who used to be so reasonable, as she often dominated conversations with her "preachy" concerns about toxins, vaccines, and cancer. Her refusal to consider other viewpoints or moderate her stance led to conflicts and estrangement, resulting in social isolation. Feeling misunderstood and unsupported, Julia sought validation within like-minded communities, creating a feedback loop where her radical beliefs were continuously reinforced.

Following a severe fallout with a childhood friend who expressed concern about her mental health, Julia somewhat reluctantly sought therapy. She frankly had hoped that therapy would be confirmation that her views were reasonable and that the rest of the world was in denial. Although the therapist was accepting and nonjudgmental, she also sought to help Julia find a deeper reason for her conspiracy-mindedness.

Eventually, in therapy, Julia addressed her unresolved grief over her mother's death and explored the emotions she had been experiencing. Through cognitive-behavioral therapy, she worked on identifying and challenging cognitive distortions that contributed to her radicalization, addressing her catastrophic and black-and-white thinking. Psychoeducation provided her with an understanding of the psychological impact of grief and the dangers of confirmation bias. She was encouraged to rebuild relationships with friends and family members, learning communication strategies to express her concerns less confrontationally and to listen to and respect differing viewpoints. Mindfulness meditation and stress reduction exercises helped her manage anxiety and obsessive thoughts about environmental and vaccine toxins.

Over time, Julia found a balance between her environmental concerns and maintaining healthy relationships. She remained active in environmental advocacy but adopted a more moderate and evidence-based approach. Her relationships with friends and family improved as she learned to communicate more effectively and consider a wider range of perspectives. Therapy eventually helped Julia understand the link between her grief and her radicalization, allowing her to address her emotional needs in healthier ways. Although she did not change most of her political beliefs, including inaccuracies regarding vaccinations, her approach to others became more compassionate and accepting.

Collective Trauma and Grieving

Beyond individual bereavement, collective trauma and historical losses can engender complicated societal grief reactions. Marginalized communities affected by systemic injustice, oppression and mass violence often carry a heavy burden of intergenerational grief (Brave Heart, 2003). Some authors describe how unresolved collective grief can be transmitted across generations, shaping group identity, memory and behavior. Unacknowledged historical trauma can fuel social unrest, extremist ideation, and cycles of retaliatory violence (Hirschberger, 2018).

Political scientist Judith Butler (2020) examines how grief can be exploited for the "instrumentalization of affect to wage wars and disrupt democratic processes" (p. 70). Stoking rage and fear about the erosion of cultural identity and way of life is a common tactic of far-right populist movements. A sense of "aggrieved entitlement" over lost status and privilege can drive reactionary backlash (Kimmel, 2017). Paradoxically, dominant groups in society may feel victimized by perceived threats to their power and resort to extremism to defend it.

Extremist groups may also exploit people's grief and emotional vulnerabilities for radicalization and recruitment (Webber & Kruglanski, 2017). Intense feelings of anger, humiliation, uncertainty, and powerlessness can make simplistic ideological narratives and solutions seem appealing (Kruglanski et al., 2014). Young people grieving lost relationships, communities, or a sense of self may be especially vulnerable to extremists offering belonging and purpose (Campelo, Oppetit, Neau, Cohen, & Bronsard, 2018).

Mason (2018) argues that growing partisan polarization is less about policy differences and more about conflicting social identities, grievances, and emotions. In a climate of "affective polarization," politics becomes deeply personal, and the other side is viewed with anger and distrust instead of civil disagreement (Iyengar, Lelkes, Levendusky, Malhotra, & Westwood, 2019). Partisan moral convictions, tribalism, and demonization of the other increasingly guide beliefs and behaviors (Finkel et al., 2020). Politically moderate people may be grieving the loss of civility and long for a return to a time when politics were more concerned with policy differences and topic focused discussions and debates. Initiating discussions about poverty, immigration, foreign policy, and other political topics can quickly become contentious and overly emotional with acquaintances or family members who have become polarized politically.

Online algorithms can create echo chambers and "filter bubbles" that isolate people in silos of grievance and fear, accelerating polarization (Ribeiro, Ottoni, West, Almeida, & Meira, 2020). Emotionally arousing content provokes anger and reinforces victimhood narratives. Personal losses are reframed in terms of group oppression and existential threat. Over time, at-risk people may come to see extreme actions as justifiable, even necessary, to defend the in-group and express pain.

As we argued in Chapter 2, the tendency to see one's perspective as correct is all but inherent in human nature. Haidt (2012) argues that ideological "group think" and the impulse to defend one's moral tribe are rooted in evolutionary adaptations for cooperation. In a polarized political environment, the social incentives for partisan conformity and punishment of deviance are strong. Dissent or openness to the other side's perspective can be seen as a betrayal, risking a loss of social standing and support. Constrained by these dynamics, people struggling with grief may find it difficult to process their emotions authentically and connect with others who don't share their partisan identity.

The following case of Emily illustrates how belief in a collective trauma can have a negative impact on life.

> Emily, a 26-year-old Caucasian woman and part-time college student, sought counseling with one of the authors due to an online gambling problem, a habit she said she had acquired with the man she was dating. She also reported increasing anxiety, anger, and a sense of disconnection from her

family and friends. Emily grew up in a very small, predominantly white town that had experienced significant economic decline over the past few decades. Many residents, including Emily's parents, had lost their jobs due to a mill's closures and felt left behind by the rapidly changing world.

Emily grew up wretchedly poor, more so than most of the other poor families in her town. She went to a public school where the narrative had been that the poverty around her was due to the devastation in the American South from the Civil War. She had been raised with the "Lost Cause" myth, a historical narrative that emerged in the southern United States after the Civil War. This interpretation of history, reiterated in her school classes and at her church, portrayed the Confederate cause as heroic and justified, while downplaying or denying the central role of slavery in the conflict and the cruelty inflicted on Black people during this time.

During therapy sessions, Emily expressed a deep sense of loss and nostalgia for a past she had never known—a time when her community was thriving, and people like her family were respected and secure. She spoke of the "good old days" when traditional values were upheld, and the town's cultural identity was strong. She stated that her goal was to move to a place where segregation was the norm and women could be "traditional-classy … and no online gambling, naturally!" Yet her world view was even more reactionary than it seemed.

As Emily entered her late teenage years, she became increasingly interested in far-right populist movements online. While her peers were interested in dating, pop culture, sports, or experiences of faith, Emily was attracted to an angry side of the world that she felt explained the emptiness she felt. She found solace in online communities that echoed her feelings of grief, anger, and resentment toward the perceived erosion of her cultural identity and way of life. These groups provided a sense of belonging and purpose, offering simplistic explanations for the complex socio-economic issues her community faced.

Through her interactions with these online communities, Emily began to adopt an "us vs. them" mentality, viewing those with different political beliefs or sexual orientations as threats to her group's identity and existence. In time her views became overtly racist. She expressed a sense of aggrieved entitlement, feeling that her community had been wronged and that they were justified in taking extreme measures to defend their way of life. Eventually, she began dating someone that she met in an online group and became even more vehement in her beliefs. When they were not gambling or smoking marijuana, they spent time affiliating with like-minded people.

As Emily became more engrossed in these echo chambers, her relationships with family and friends who held more moderate views began to deteriorate.

She found herself arguing with loved ones, accusing them of betraying their "white heritage" and siding with the "Jewish enemy." The algorithms of the online platforms she used reinforced her beliefs, exposing her to increasingly extreme content that validated her fears and anger, as well as providing an excuse for her aggrieved lifestyle.

The echo chambers and filter bubbles created by online algorithms further accelerated Emily's radicalization process, isolating her from diverse perspectives and reinforcing her sense of grievance. As her partisan moral convictions grew stronger, Emily began to view those with different beliefs as morally inferior, leading to a breakdown in her relationships and an inability to process her emotions in a healthy manner.

At one point Emily was taken to a psychiatric nurse practitioner by her mother and diagnosed as paranoid. She was given antipsychotic medications, which did little to dampen her enthusiasm for rural white extremists.

Emily's case, quite remarkable for a young woman, illustrates how collective trauma and unresolved grief can be exploited by extremist groups to radicalize vulnerable individuals. The sense of loss and nostalgia for a perceived golden age, coupled with feelings of resentment and victimhood, made Emily susceptible to the simplistic narratives offered by far-right populist movements.

Through therapy, Emily began to explore the underlying grief and trauma that fueled her attraction to extremist ideologies. By addressing her feelings of loss, resentment, and powerlessness in a safe and nonjudgmental environment, Emily slowly began to develop a more balanced understanding of her experiences and the complex socio-political issues her community faced. She now believes that her history of gambling and drugs were dangerous distractions, a pernicious form of self-medication, keeping her from feeling her true grief.

Tribalism as a Source of Grief

While partisanship can be used to escape personal or social grief, partisan conflict can also serve as a source of grief. Partisan feelings, characterized by solid allegiance to a particular political party or ideology, can themselves be a source of grief and loss when they negatively affect interpersonal relationships (Mason, 2018). The emotional investment in political identities and beliefs can strain relationships, causing painful conflicts with friends and family.

One reason for this is taught in almost every introductory psychology class. Cognitive dissonance theory suggests that people experience psychological discomfort when confronted with information or opinions that contradict their beliefs (Festinger, 1957). To reduce this discomfort, they may dismiss opposing views or avoid discussions with those who hold different opinions. This defensive posture can lead to strained relationships and a sense of isolation.

Additionally, partisan feelings are often accompanied by strong emotions like anger, frustration, and even hatred toward perceived political opponents (Iyengar & Westwood, 2015). When political beliefs are tied to religious and moral convictions, disagreements are viewed as not just intellectual debates but moral confrontations. This makes reconciliation difficult and contributes to emotional distress, especially when these feelings are projected onto others.

One of the most immediate manifestations of partisan-related grief is damaged or lost relationships. Friends and family members may distance themselves or cut ties to avoid constant conflict (Pew Research Center, 2017). This relational loss can be profoundly painful, representing the erosion of support systems and shared histories. It can evoke feelings of sadness, anger, isolation and helplessness. Examples are when longtime friends fail to contact each other because of political differences. A more poignant example, the case of John, follows.

When John first contacted a therapist, he was sitting in his living room, holding a framed photograph of his mother. He had been crying for hours. The news of her passing had hit him harder than he expected, considering the tumultuous relationship they had shared throughout his life. As a middle-aged, politically moderate man, John could not figure out why she constantly attacked his morals and, mostly, his politics.

Looking back, John realized that their differences had created a rift between them, leading to a sense of emotional distance and alienation. He had always felt misunderstood and judged by his mother, who seemingly disapproved of his choices and values. This did not make any sense to him since they went to the same denomination of church, and he considered himself even more religious than her. The hurt, frustration, and rejection he had experienced over the years had left a deep scar on his heart.

John initially blamed himself for these differences. He had self-identified that he was on the autism spectrum, later confirmed by a psychologist. He believed that his occasional lack of social skills was a chronic annoyance to his mother and was the source of his problems with her.

Eventually, John began to see that he was not the only instigator of difficulties with his mother. He could make more sense of their relationship if they had disagreed about religion or even his choice of careers. That was common where he came from and somehow seemed more reasonable and acceptable. However, they had always disagreed over things of minimal importance to him, like who was elected in local elections, and what they stood for. While his father was alive, his mother was less open about these differences. But when her husband died, she seemed to lose restraint, sarcastically commenting on his "irresponsible" liberal values, which were actually mainstream. For a time, John quit posting on social media, hoping that it would give his mother a reduced target to criticize him.

When his mother's health began to decline, John put away his anxiety and reached out, offering to move her into his house so he could assist in taking care of her. It was a gesture of compassion and love, a desire to put aside their differences and ensure her well-being. However, his mother angrily refused, and John couldn't help but feel that her decision was influenced by her long-standing perception of him as too liberal. The rejection had stung, leaving him feeling helpless and grieving for the relationship they could have had.

John pretended that their disagreement was due to her age. He looked for an excuse based on her declining cognitive status or poor health. However, he had to face the truth. The differences between them became apparent in his youth. He saw her as racist, sexist, and mean spirited to people different than herself. Her age had little to do with these lifelong traits.

Now, as he sat with the weight of her loss, John found himself grappling with a complex array of emotions. The grief and sorrow of losing a parent, regardless of their differences, washed over him in waves. He felt a deep sense of regret and guilt, wondering if he could have done more to bridge the gap between them, to convince her to accept his help. Shouldn't he have lied to her? Perhaps pretended to be less moderate than he was? The lost opportunities for connection and reconciliation haunted him.

At the same time, John couldn't help but feel anger and resentment toward his mother. He struggled to understand how she could have let their political differences, as strange as hers seemed to him, come between them, even in her final years. The frustration of their strained relationship lingered, unresolved and raw.

As he thought about his feelings, John realized that his mother's passing had left him with a sense of emotional incompleteness, along with guilt, and deep shame. The issues that had plagued their relationship remained unresolved, leaving him yearning for closure. He knew that he would need to find a way to come to terms with these feelings, to find peace within himself. He hoped that therapy would be a solution.

At its core, political tribalism represents an unwavering loyalty to one's political faction, often at the expense of other dimensions of identity. This allegiance can become so integral to one's sense of self that it overshadows familial bonds, leading to estrangement and conflict. Families, traditionally a source of support and love, are not immune to the divisive forces of political tribalism. The dinner table, once a place for shared meals and stories, has, in some households, become a battleground for ideological disputes. These divisions can strain relationships to the breaking point, transforming gatherings meant for connection into occasions of tension and discord. When the loss is permanent, sometimes the grief seems irreconcilable.

Disenfranchised Grief

Disenfranchised grief occurs when a loss is not recognized or validated by society (Doka, 1989). In the context of partisan conflict, the grief over damaged relationships and social discord is often dismissed or minimized, as political disagreements are seen as common or inevitable. This lack of acknowledgment can intensify the grieving process and compound feelings of alienation. In an "us vs. them" political climate, people may feel unable to express vulnerable emotions without being judged as disloyal to their ideological tribe.

This case study illustrates how political partisanship, and significant electoral outcomes can profoundly affect an individual's mental health, highlighting the intersection between political identity and psychological well-being. The case of Alex illustrates this.

Alex is a 45-year-old man residing in a suburban neighborhood. He works as a university staff member in a private school and has been actively involved in local politics for many years. Alex identifies strongly with conservative values. The 2020 US Presidential election was particularly significant for him due to the highly polarized political climate and the implications he believed it had for the future of the country.

Leading up to the 2020 Presidential election, Alex was deeply invested in the campaign, attending rallies, engaging in heated discussions online, and even volunteering for his preferred candidate's campaign. He perceived the election as a critical turning point, with the outcome determining not just policy directions but the very fabric of American society.

When the results were announced and it became clear that his candidate had lost, Alex was devastated. He felt a profound sense of loss, almost as if a loved one had died. This grief was not just about the political defeat but was intertwined with his identity and vision for the future. Alex experienced a range of emotions including shock, disbelief, anger, and deep sadness.

Initially, Alex couldn't believe the results. He spent hours consuming news and social media content, hoping for a different outcome or some form of reversal. This denial phase prolonged his acceptance of reality.

Alex's grief soon morphed into anger. He blamed various factors including media bias, electoral fraud claims, and even friends and family members who voted differently. This anger often resulted in heated arguments and strained relationships. Alex eventually began endorsing several alternative theories regarding the election, some of which were extremely unlikely.

As weeks passed, Alex's anger subsided into a deep sadness. He became withdrawn, avoided social activities, and isolated himself from friends and family. His work performance suffered, and he experienced difficulty sleeping and a loss of appetite. The election loss led Alex to question his place in the country he once felt deeply connected to. He struggled with feelings of powerlessness and a loss of purpose, leading to an angry crisis about his role and beliefs.

At his wife's insistence, Alex sought counseling to discuss his grief and its impact on his mental health. In therapy, Alex worked through his emotions, focusing on acknowledging that his grief was legitimate, and understanding its depth helped Alex feel less isolated in his experience.

Over time, Alex began to heal from his profound grief. He re-engaged with his social network, resumed hobbies he once enjoyed, and found a balanced way to stay informed and involved in politics without compromising his well-being. His journey through grief highlighted the profound impact of political events on mental health and the importance of seeking support during such challenging times. He never changed his core beliefs or his opinion that the election had been stolen. However, those beliefs no longer put a wedge between him and others.

The Role of Mental Health Professionals

As clinicians, we play a vital role in supporting clients experiencing grief, whether due to personal loss or political and social divisions. By providing a safe, nonjudgmental space to process the full spectrum of grief-related emotions, we can help mitigate the lure of extremism and foster healthy coping.

A key priority is validating grief and anger and exploring underlying vulnerabilities without judgment. As Lamia (2022) emphasizes, anger and shame are both a natural part of grieving and should be met with care rather than pathologized. At the same time, we must be prepared to firmly challenge destructive thoughts and behaviors. Structured therapies for prolonged grief reactions, such as complicated grief therapy, can help clients find meaningful ways to connect with loss, develop coping skills, and reconstruct identity (Shear, 2015).

With grief related to partisan divisions, acknowledging the significance of the loss is essential. Damaged relationships and the social fabric are actual, painful losses that deserve to be mourned. Clients need space to grieve the disconnection, disenchantment, or betrayal they may feel regarding political identities and systems of meaning. Exploring how identity and moral values shape these emotions can yield insight and self-compassion.

Cultivating flexibility and acceptance of ambiguity are key treatment goals. Lamia (2022) recommends helping grieving clients find "shades of gray," building capacity for cognitive flexibility and more contextual thinking. Mindfulness practices, self-regulation skills, and expressive arts can provide healthy outlets and ease rigid reactivity (Thompson & Neimeyer, 2014). Over time, clients may move toward a more integrated, less defensive sense of self capable of engaging with differences and coping with their feelings.

In cases of more severe ideological rigidity and us vs. them thinking, cognitive restructuring and direct exposure to different perspectives may be warranted. Carefully unpacking beliefs about grievance and entitlement with Socratic questioning can introduce doubt and curb the appeal of extremist narratives. With sufficient stabilization, some clients may benefit from structured dialogue with those of differing views to build empathy and reduce hostility (Bruneau & Saxe, 2012).

At the same time, we need discernment about when cross-divide engagement could be counterproductive or unsafe. People in the acute throes of extremist perspectives may not be psychologically ready for such exposure. Here, strengthening life-affirming coping skills, social support, and self-efficacy is the priority. Restoring a bereaved person's sense of agency and connection is vital in resolving grief and loosening the grip of rigid ideologies. When appropriate, referral to specialized programs for preventing and intervening in radicalization processes may be advised.

On a broader scale, mental health professionals can advocate for policies, programs, and civic dialogues that address the psychosocial roots of polarization and extremism (Weine, Eisenman, Kinsler, Glik, & Polutnik, 2017). By educating the public about the links between grief, ideology, and social cohesion, we can help shift the conversation and reduce stigma. Consulting with schools, faith communities, and other local institutions to build resilience and reconciliation skills can help mend the social fabric. Ultimately, by attending to individual and collective grief with wisdom and care, we can contribute to a society of greater understanding and compassion across differences.

Summary

In a time of profound disruption and polarization, the interplay between grief and political identities is complex and consequential. Unresolved grief can make people vulnerable to the rigid certainties of extreme ideologies. At the same time, entrenched partisan conflicts are themselves a source of widespread grief as relationships and social trust fray.

While these dynamics can feed a grim cycle of division and despair, they need not have the last word. In spaces of therapeutic support and public conversation alike, grief and vulnerability can be powerful points of connection. By having the courage to acknowledge loss together, we may begin to rediscover our common humanity.

References

Berger, J. M. (2018). *Extremism*. Boston: MIT Press.

Bonanno, G. A., & Kaltman, S. (2001). The varieties of grief experience. *Clinical Psychology Review*, *21*(5), 705–734.

Brave Heart, M. Y. (2003). The historical trauma response among natives and its relationship with substance abuse: A Lakota illustration. *Journal of Psychoactive Drugs*, *35*(1),7–13. doi: 10.1080/02791072.2003.10399988. PMID: 12733753.

Bruneau, E. G., & Saxe, R. (2012). The power of being heard: The benefits of 'perspective-giving' in the context of intergroup conflict. *Journal of Experimental Social Psychology*, *48*(4), 855–866.

Butler, J. (2020). *The force of nonviolence: An ethico-political bind.* London: Verso Books.

Campelo, N., Oppetit, A., Neau, F., Cohen, D., & Bronsard, G. (2018). Who are the European youths willing to engage in radicalization? A multidisciplinary review of their psychological and social profiles. *European Psychiatry*, *52*, 1–14.

Doka, K. J. (1989). *Disenfranchised grief: Recognizing hidden sorrow*. Lanham, MD: Lexington Books.

Festinger, L. (1957). *A theory of cognitive dissonance*. Redwood City: Stanford University Press.

Finkel, E. J., Bail, C. A., Cikara, M., Ditto, P. H., Iyengar, S., Klar, S., Mason, L., et al. (2020). Political sectarianism in America. *Science*, *370*(6516), 533–536.

Haidt, J. (2012). *The righteous mind: Why good people are divided by politics and religion*. New York, NY: Vintage.

Hirschberger, G. (2018). Collective trauma and the social construction of meaning. *Frontiers in Psychology*, *9*, 1441.

Hogg, M. A. (2014). From uncertainty to extremism: Social categorization and identity processes. *Current Directions in Psychological Science*, *23(5)*, 338–342.

Iyengar, S., & Westwood, S. J. (2015). Fear and loathing across party lines: New evidence on group polarization. *American Journal of Political Science*, *59*(3), 690–707.

Iyengar, S., Lelkes, Y., Levendusky, M., Malhotra, N., & Westwood, S. J. (2019). The origins and consequences of affective polarization in the United States. *Annual Review of Political Science*, *22*, 129–146.

Janoff-Bulman, R. (1992). *Shattered assumptions: Towards a new psychology of trauma*. New York, NY: Free Press.

Kimmel, M. (2017). *Angry white men: American masculinity at the end of an era*. London: Hachette UK.

Kruglanski, A. W., Gelfand, M. J., Bélanger, J. J., Sheveland, A., Hetiarachchi, M., & Gunaratna, R. (2014). The psychology of radicalization and deradicalization: How significant quest impacts violent extremism. *Political Psychology*, *35*, 69–93.

Kübler-Ross, E. (1974). *Questions and answers on death and dying*. New York, NY: Macmillan.

Lamia, M. C. (2022). *Grief isn't something to get over*. Washington, DC: American Psychological Association Press.

Mancini, A. D. (2019). When acute grief morphs into PTSD: Understanding the effects of loss in the aftermath of mass shootings and other tragedies. *Traumatology, 25*(4), 277–281.

Mason, L. (2018). *Uncivil agreement: How politics became our identity*. University of Chicago Press.

Neimeyer, R. A. (2019). Meaning reconstruction in bereavement: Development of a research program. *Death Studies, 43*(2), 79–91.

Pew Research Center. (2017). *The partisan divide on political values grows even wider*. Pew Research Center.

Prigerson, H. G., Kakarala, S., Gang, J., & Maciejewski, P. K. (2021). History and status of prolonged grief disorder as a psychiatric diagnosis. *Annual Review of Clinical Psychology, 17*, 109–126.

Ribeiro, M. H., Ottoni, R., West, R., Almeida, V. A., & Meira, W. (2020). Auditing radicalization pathways on YouTube. In *Proceedings of the 2020 Conference on Fairness, Accountability, and Transparency* (pp. 131–141).

Shear, M. K. (2012). Grief and mourning gone awry: Pathway and course of complicated grief. *Dialogues in Clinical Neuroscience, 14*(2), 119–128.

Thompson, B. E., & Neimeyer, R. A. (Eds.) (2014). *Grief and the expressive arts: Practices for creating meaning*. New York, NY: Routledge.

Webber, D., & Kruglanski, A. W. (2017). Psychological factors in radicalization: A "3 N" approach. In G. LaFree & J. D. Freilich (Eds.), *The handbook of the criminology of terrorism* (pp. 33–46). New York, NY: Wiley & Sons.

Weine, S., Eisenman, D. P., Kinsler, J., Glik, D. C., & Polutnik, C. (2017). Addressing violent extremism as public health policy and practice. *Behavioral Sciences of Terrorism and Political Aggression, 9*(3), 208–221.

8

COMPLEX DISORDERS AND POLITICS

Personality and Politics: When Extremes Intersect

In the current sociopolitical landscape, characterized by intense polarization and heated partisan anger, therapists face a unique challenge. They must distinguish between symptoms of mental health disorders and characteristics of extreme political partisanship. Following qualitative interviews, detailed in Appendix A, we asked 184 practitioners to identify which diagnoses were likely to be associated with extreme liberals and which were likely to be related to extreme conservatives. We then compared these findings with nonpartisan clients. The results, however, were not particularly illuminating. The data revealed that if a therapist tended to see trauma patients, then their clients, whether on the left or the right, were primarily drawn from that population. Similarly, if a therapist specialized in treating anxiety or depression, their patients were likely to be anxious or depressed, irrespective of their political leanings. There was no significant difference between the frequencies of these conditions on the left or the right compared to a therapist's expected base rate.

However, when we asked therapists to identify *which diagnoses were the most challenging to treat* in highly partisan individuals, a clearer pattern emerged. Therapists consistently pointed to specific diagnoses as particularly problematic when dealing with clients with strong political affiliations. Similarly, when we inquired about which diagnoses were likely to present with partisan sentiments that potentially masked deeper issues, there was a discernible pattern. Interestingly, five of the same diagnoses were repeated in both categories, suggesting a significant overlap.

DOI: 10.4324/9781032651217-8

Several conditions warrant attention in this context, including borderline personality disorder (BPD), bipolar disorder, narcissistic personality disorder (NPD), histrionic personality disorder (HPD), antisocial personality disorder (ASPD), and paranoid personality disorder (PPD). Beyond specific diagnoses, therapists noted that many individuals who are the most difficult to treat possess particular characteristics that extend beyond their diagnoses. These characteristics often include rigid thinking, an inability to consider alternative viewpoints, and a propensity for viewing the world in a black-and-white manner. Many are angry, perhaps motivated by deep feelings of shame and fear. Such traits can complicate the therapeutic process of a highly partisan client or anyone, making it challenging for therapists to help these clients achieve meaningful progress.

This chapter explores the relationship between these mental health conditions and political partisanship, the consequences of misdiagnosis, and the role of the therapist in navigating this complex terrain. These challenges are not merely about the presence of a particular condition but are deeply intertwined with the individual's inflexible worldview and entrenched beliefs. This rigidity can hinder the therapeutic alliance, limit the effectiveness of interventions in the therapy space, and ultimately affect overall treatment outcomes.

Borderline Personality Disorder

In Chapter 1, we remarked on how people with BPD may be similar to highly partisan people. The borderline analogy is often a helpful metaphor because people with BPD and those who are highly partisan share several key characteristics that can make differentiation challenging. As discussed in Chapter 1, one of the most prominent similarities is the tendency to engage in splitting, a cognitive distortion characterized by black-and-white thinking (Ward, Benjamin, & Zimmerman, 2022). In the political context, this manifests as viewing one's side as inherently good and righteous while perceiving the opposing side as evil, venal, and morally corrupt. This polarized worldview not only hinders constructive political discourse but also mirrors the instability in self-image and relationships observed in BPD.

Another parallel between BPD and extreme partisanship is heightened emotional reactivity and identity instability (Kockler et al., 2022). Both groups may exhibit intense emotional responses to events, discussions, or figures that challenge their beliefs. This emotional volatility can lead to interpersonal conflicts and strained relationships, as the reactive nature often overshadows rational analysis and dialogue. To complicate diagnosis and treatment, people with BPD and those who are highly partisan often anchor their identity to their beliefs, perceiving any challenge to these beliefs as a personal attack. This fusion of individual identity with political ideology can lead to rigidity of thought and a reluctance to consider alternative viewpoints.

Some highly partisan people, in fact, do have borderline traits or a full-blown disorder. The attraction of people with BPD to extremist political groups can be understood through several psychological factors. These groups provide a clear sense of identity and purpose, which appeals to the emotional vulnerability and need for belonging experienced by those with BPD. The polarized rhetoric and us vs. them narratives align with the dichotomous thinking style characteristic of BPD, making these ideologies feel relatable and attractive. Moreover, the impulsivity associated with BPD can find an outlet in the excitement and urgency of radical political activities.

The involvement of individuals with BPD in politically extreme groups can have profound implications for their interpersonal relationships. As they become more entrenched in polarizing ideologies, family and friends may find themselves increasingly alienated by the individual's extreme political views. Communication breakdown and a lack of empathy can strain these relationships, as the us vs. them mentality adopted by the individual spills over into personal interactions.

Furthermore, the impulsivity and risk-taking behaviors associated with BPD, when combined with the aggressive tactics often employed by extremist groups, can lead to situations that jeopardize the safety and well-being of the individual and those around them. This can cause significant distress and concern for loved ones, further straining interpersonal bonds.

The following is an example of a person with BPD who can be said to have used politics to express borderline traits.

LYNETTE: RELIGION, POLITICS, AND BORDERLINE FUNCTIONING

Lynette is a 52-year-old woman whose life has been marked by a repetitive and destructive pattern within conservative Evangelical churches, reflecting her intertwined religious and political beliefs. Lynette's history with conservative Evangelical churches began in her early thirties following a history of eating disorder, substance abuse, and multiple suicide attempts.

Drawn to strict Fundamentalist doctrinal teachings and their congregations, she found a sense of belonging and purpose that seemed to keep her most pernicious symptoms at bay. However, Lynette's involvement in these communities has repeatedly ended in turmoil and division.

Lynette's engagement with each church she has joined follows a predictable pattern that plays out over many months. Initially, she presents herself as a devout and enthusiastic member, often taking on leadership roles within Bible study groups or church committees. Her enthusiasm, Christian testimony, and apparent dedication earn her the trust and admiration of many congregants.

Over time, however, Lynette begins to introduce subtle criticisms and doubts about the church's direction and leadership. She adeptly identifies existing fissures within the congregation and exacerbates them, aligning herself with one faction while demonizing the other. Her skill in manipulating church politics, which appears to operate unconsciously for her, becomes evident as she gradually sows seeds of discord.

Lynette's religious beliefs are inextricably linked to her political ideology. She advocates for a strict, literal interpretation of the Bible, which aligns with her ultra-conservative political views. Her rhetoric often includes a mix of religious fervor and political extremism, portraying any deviation from her beliefs as a betrayal of actual Christian values. This blend of religion and politics makes Lynette a polarizing figure. Her insistence that the church must take stronger stances on political issues, such as abortion and denial of LGBTQ and women's rights, alienates those with more moderate views, even people who are otherwise conservative. She frames these issues in stark, moralistic terms, creating a binary worldview where her side is righteous, and the other is sinful. This includes the "sinners" people in her church, who she views as somehow failing the Lord. This process may unfold over many months or even years and Lynette is entirely unaware that she is repeating a pattern that she has followed with many other congregations

As Lynette's influence grows, so does the tension within the congregation. Disagreements escalate into open conflicts, with members taking sides. Lynette's faction often feels validated in their beliefs, encouraged by her passionate leadership and spiritual commitment. The opposing faction, meanwhile, feels increasingly marginalized and criticized.

Eventually, the church reaches a breaking point. The once cohesive community becomes fractured, with trust eroded and relationships damaged. At this juncture, Lynette typically departs, citing the church's "deep, sinful failure" to meet her spiritual needs and accusing it of not being sufficiently Biblical. Typically, she frames her departure as a moral high ground, reinforcing her self-image as a defender of true faith and conservative values.

Lynette's departure from the church does not mark the end of the cycle. Shortly after leaving, she finds another conservative Evangelical congregation, perhaps with a slightly different doctrine. Over time, she will repeat the same pattern of behavior. Her presence, initially seen as joyous and positive, becomes a toxic catalyst for conflict, and her departure leaves a trail of division and disarray.

Lynette's behavior can be understood through the lens of personality disorders, particularly those characterized by manipulative and divisive tendencies. Her actions suggest traits commonly associated with BPD. Her need for admiration, coupled with a lack of empathy, drives her to create conflicts where she can play a central, controlling role, also suggesting touches of narcissism.

Additionally, her black-and-white thinking and intense fear of abandonment may contribute to her need to constantly test the loyalty of those around her. By creating divisions and then leaving, she ensures that she remains the focal point of drama and attention, even in her absence.

Addressing the intersection of BPD and high political partisanship requires an approach that focuses on both the underlying personality disorder and the individual's attraction to extreme ideologies. Psychotherapy, particularly Dialectical Behavior Therapy (DBT), has shown promise in treating BPD by teaching skills for emotional regulation, distress tolerance, and interpersonal effectiveness (Swales, 2019). By helping individuals manage their intense emotions and impulsivity, DBT can reduce the appeal of extreme political groups and improve overall functioning.

In addition to addressing the core symptoms of BPD, it is almost always valuable to foster open communication, empathy, and understanding within the individual's social network. Family and friends can play a vital role in providing a supportive environment that encourages the individual to explore their beliefs and values in a nonjudgmental manner. By maintaining a connection and showing genuine concern, loved ones can help the individual feel less isolated and more receptive to alternative perspectives. Through a combination of psychotherapy, emotional regulation skills training, and fostering empathy and understanding within social networks, people with BPD can be better equipped to manage their emotions, maintain healthier relationships, and develop a more subtle understanding of the political landscape.

Narcissistic Personality Disorder and Political Partisanship

NPD presents another challenge in the realm of political partisanship. People with NPD often exhibit a grandiose sense of self-importance, a need for admiration, and a lack of empathy (Swales, Clark, & Farnam, 2024). These traits can manifest in the political sphere in ways that resemble hyper-partisanship but are driven by different underlying motivations.

People with NPD are often charismatic and may be drawn to the spotlight that political involvement can provide. They may express solid political opinions and align themselves with a particular party or ideology. However, their steadfast commitment to these views may be superficial, as their primary goal is to gain attention, admiration, and validation from others. Some Internet and media figures may seem to fit this description as they bounce around the ideological spectrum until they find a supportive, adoring audience who they can attempt to impress with their self-assumed brilliance.

One of the hallmarks of NPD is a sense of entitlement and a belief in one's superiority (Elleuch, 2024). In the political context, this can manifest as an unwavering conviction in the righteousness of their beliefs and dismissal of opposing viewpoints. However, unlike people with genuine political convictions, those with NPD may be more likely to shift their allegiances if doing so serves their ego needs as sometimes occurs with political candidates.

People with NPD may also exploit political causes or movements for personal gain, using them as vehicles to enhance their status and influence. They may seek leadership positions or high-profile roles within political organizations, not out of a genuine commitment to the cause but as a means to garner attention and admiration.

In treatment, therapists must recognize that the political views expressed by those with NPD may not reflect deeply held beliefs but rather serve as instruments for ego gratification. Attempting to challenge or modify these views directly may be counterproductive, as the individual's attachment to these views is rooted in their personality structure rather than genuine political conviction. Instead, treatment for NPD in the context of political partisanship should focus on addressing the core traits and patterns of the disorder. This may involve helping the individual develop greater self-awareness, empathy, and the ability to form genuine connections with others. By addressing these underlying issues, therapists can help people with NPD build a more stable sense of self that is less reliant on external validation and more capable of engaging in authentic political discourse.

Histrionic Personality Disorder and Political Partisanship

A pattern of excessive emotionality and attention-seeking behavior characterizes HPD. People with HPD often exhibit a strong desire to be the center of attention, engage in provocative or seductive behavior, and have a rapidly shifting and shallow expression of emotions (Magid & Fox, 2022). These traits can manifest in the political sphere in ways that may be misinterpreted as genuine political fervor or hyper-partisanship.

People with HPD may be drawn to the drama and intensity of high-level partisan political causes. The polarized nature of these movements provides many opportunities for people with HPD to express their emotions, seek attention, and engage in provocative behavior. They may become deeply involved in political activism, not necessarily due to a genuine commitment to the cause, but because it allows them to be in the spotlight and elicit reactions from others.

The rapidly shifting emotions and dramatic expressions characteristic of HPD can be mistaken for enthusiastic political convictions. People with HPD may express strong, seemingly unwavering opinions on political issues. Still, these opinions may be shallow and easily swayed by the reactions of others or the potential for attention. They may jump from one extreme position to another, not due to a change in beliefs, but because a new position offers a fresh opportunity for attention and drama.

In the context of political partisanship, people with HPD may engage in provocative or seductive behavior to gain attention and influence within their chosen political group. They may use their sexuality or physical appearance to draw attention to themselves and their political views, blurring the lines between genuine political engagement and attention-seeking behavior.

For those with HPD, the intense emotions and sense of belonging associated with extreme political groups can be particularly appealing. The us vs. them mentality and the high stakes often associated with partisan causes provide a stage upon which they can express their emotions and seek validation from others who share their views.

In treatment, therapists need to recognize that the political engagement of clients with HPD may be primarily driven by their personality traits rather than deeply held political beliefs (Babl et al., 2022). Challenging their political views directly may be counterproductive, as it may be experienced as a threat to their sense of self and their need for attention. Instead, treatment should focus on helping those with HPD develop a more stable sense of self, learn to regulate their emotions and build genuine relationships based on mutual understanding and respect (Babl et al., 2022). This may involve teaching skills for self-reflection, emotional regulation, and interpersonal communication. By addressing the core features of HPD, therapists can help these clients develop a more authentic sense of self and engage in political discourse in a manner that is less driven by attention-seeking and more grounded in genuine beliefs and values.

SARAH

Sarah was a middle-aged woman who was treated by one of the authors many years ago.

She presented with both histrionic and narcissistic personality features. From an early age, Sarah exhibited a pattern of selfishness, self-admiration, excessive emotionality and attention-seeking behavior, often displaying inappropriate seductive or provocative behaviors in a variety of contexts.

In her young adulthood, Sarah was initially drawn to left-wing political activism, where she found an outlet for her tendencies toward self-dramatization and exaggerated need for positive attention. She engaged in flamboyant, theatrical behaviors during protests and rallies, which garnered her significant attention and a devoted following, thus reinforcing her dysfunctional patterns.

However, Sarah's political beliefs appeared to lack depth and stability, likely due to the lack of a coherent sense of self that is characteristic of both HPD and narcissistic traits. When a right-wing movement emerged that valued provocative and politically incorrect speech, Sarah made a dramatic public shift in her allegiances. This sudden transformation brought her local attention, satisfying her narcissistic need for admiration and grandiosity.

As Sarah's public profile grew, her behavior became increasingly extreme and polarizing. She exhibited the selfish behavior and lack of empathy often seen in NPD, demonizing her former allies and constructing a grandiose narrative around her political conversion. She was quick to sell out even her friends if it meant more attention and praise. Her histrionic tendencies were evident in her constant need for stimulation and her embellished, attention-grabbing stories about her past.

From a clinical perspective, Sarah's case illustrates how personality disorders can manifest in the realm of political behavior. Individuals with HPD and NPD may be drawn to extremist movements that provide a platform for their dysfunctional needs for attention, admiration, and self-dramatization. Their opinions and allegiances may shift based on what garners the most validation and reinforcement of their disordered personality traits. Social media offers those with HPD and HPD a limitless and always available stage on which to perform. Getting "likes" for their histrionic behavior becomes a constant source of gratification, which can be hard to interrupt during the therapeutic process.

In conceptualizing and treating patients like Sarah, clinicians must be attuned to the underlying psychological factors driving their dramatic political transformations and polarizing behaviors. By addressing the core emotional needs and distorted cognitions associated with HPD and NPD, therapeutic interventions may help to mitigate the impact of these personality disorders on the individual and society at large.

Antisocial Personality Disorder and Political Partisanship

ASPD is characterized by a pervasive pattern of disregard for and violation of the rights of others (Swales et al., 2024). People with ASPD often engage in deceitful, manipulative, and impulsive behaviors, lacking empathy and remorse for their actions. In the context of political partisanship, people with ASPD may be attracted to extreme causes not out of genuine belief but for the opportunity to exploit and manipulate others.

People with ASPD are often skilled at reading others and identifying vulnerabilities, as well as general deficits in the development of conscience. Often, these tendencies are evident even in adolescence (Hamlat, Young, & Hankin, 2020). They may use their charm and charisma to gain trust and influence within political groups, only to later exploit these connections for personal gain. They may express strong political opinions and engage in heated debates, not because they hold these beliefs profoundly but because they enjoy the thrill of conflict and the power that comes with manipulating others.

In the online world, those with ASPD may be particularly drawn to the anonymity and lack of consequences that the Internet provides. They may engage in trolling behavior, deliberately provoking and antagonizing others for their amusement. They may also use online platforms to spread misinformation, sow discord, and manipulate public opinion, all to cause chaos and assert their power.

Unlike other personality disorders discussed in this chapter, people with ASPD are less likely to be genuinely attracted to the ideological content of extreme political movements.

Instead, they are drawn to the opportunity for exploitation, manipulation, and the thrill of causing trouble. They may align themselves with various political causes, not out of conviction but because these groups provide a platform for their destructive behaviors.

Treating people with ASPD in the context of political partisanship is particularly challenging, as they are often resistant to change and may not see their behavior as problematic. Confrontational approaches are likely to be met with hostility and defensiveness, as people with ASPD usually view others as adversaries to be outmaneuvered rather than as allies in their personal growth.

One potential avenue for intervention is through substance abuse treatment, as people with ASPD often struggle with comorbid alcohol or drug addiction. Twelve-step programs, such as Alcoholics Anonymous or Narcotics Anonymous, can provide a structured environment where people with ASPD are held accountable for their actions and encouraged to develop empathy and concern for others. The community support and peer pressure within these groups can sometimes function as an external conscience, helping people with ASPD to regulate their behavior and consider the consequences of their actions.

It is essential to note that even with treatment, people with ASPD may continue to engage in manipulative and exploitative behaviors in the political sphere. The goal of intervention is not to change their political views but rather to help them develop a greater capacity for empathy, impulse control, and respect for the rights of others. By addressing the core features of ASPD, therapists can help these people build more authentic and prosocial relationships, both within and outside of the political realm.

Paranoid Personality Disorder, Paranoia, and Political Partisanship

PPD is characterized by a pervasive distrust and suspiciousness of others, often without sufficient basis (Lee & Santos, 2022). People with PPD may perceive benign or neutral actions as malicious, harbor unjustified doubts about the loyalty of friends and associates, and be preoccupied with conspiratorial explanations for events. These traits can manifest in the political sphere, leading to an affinity for extreme partisan views and a heightened sense of perceived threat.

Paranoia, a related but distinct concept, refers to irrational and persistent thoughts of suspicion, mistrust, and fear of others' intentions (Kapil-Pair, Landa, Hansen, Vaccaro, & Goodman, 2021). While not all people with PPD experience paranoia, and not all those with paranoid thoughts meet the criteria for PPD, the two often co-occur and can significantly influence political beliefs and behaviors.

People with PPD or paranoid tendencies may be drawn to extreme ideologies that validate their suspicions and provide a sense of certainty in an uncertain world (Stone, 2014). They may perceive political opponents as not merely misguided but as malevolent actors with hidden agendas, conspiring to undermine their way of life or strip away their rights.

For example, an individual with PPD may become fixated on the idea that a particular political party or government agency is secretly working to monitor their activities, control their thoughts, or restrict their freedoms. They may interpret innocuous events, such as a change in local ordinances or a politician's offhand remark, as evidence of a larger conspiracy. This perception of threat can lead them to align with extreme political groups that promise to defend against these perceived dangers.

The us vs. them mentality often promoted by hyper-partisan movements can be particularly appealing to those with PPD or paranoid tendencies. The clear distinction between the "good" in-group and the "evil" out-group aligns with their dichotomous thinking and provides a sense of safety and belonging. Within these groups, their suspicions and fears may be validated and even encouraged, further reinforcing their paranoid beliefs.

It is crucial to recognize that not all people with PPD or paranoid tendencies are drawn to extreme political views, and not all those with extreme political views have PPD or paranoia. As with other personality disorders, the relationship between these mental health conditions and political partisanship is complex and multifaceted.

Treating clients with PPD or paranoia in the context of political partisanship presents significant challenges. These people often have difficulty trusting others, including mental health professionals. They may view attempts to help as further evidence of a conspiracy against them. They may be resistant to treatment, believing that their suspicions are justified, and that seeking help would make them vulnerable to exploitation (Kapil-Pair et al., 2021).

Moreover, the rigid and inflexible thinking patterns associated with PPD and paranoia can make it difficult for these people to consider alternative perspectives or engage in self-reflection (Stone, 2014). As previously discussed, they may see psychotherapy as an instrument of liberals to indoctrinate others to their leftist worldviews and philosophies. Therapists may not seem liberal enough for PPD clients who espouse more extreme progressive positions, which can exacerbate suspicion and distrust. They may dismiss evidence that contradicts their beliefs and interpret challenges to their views as personal attacks.

Pharmacotherapy, such as antipsychotic medications, is rarely effective in treating PPD or paranoia, as these conditions are rooted in deeply ingrained personality traits and cognitive patterns. While medication may help manage co-occurring symptoms such as anxiety or depression, it does not address the underlying paranoid beliefs (Smith & Catanzano, 2022).

Psychotherapy, particularly cognitive-behavioral therapy (CBT), may be more effective in treating PPD and paranoia. CBT focuses on identifying and challenging irrational thoughts, developing coping strategies, and improving interpersonal skills. However, establishing trust and rapport with a therapist can be a slow and challenging process for people with these conditions. In the context of political partisanship, treatment for PPD and paranoia should focus on helping clients develop a more realistic understanding of the political landscape. This may involve gradually exposing them to diverse viewpoints, encouraging them to evaluate evidence critically, and teaching them to recognize and challenge their own cognitive biases.

Progress in treating PPD and paranoia is often slow, and many with these conditions may never seek or fully engage in treatment. The deeply ingrained nature of their beliefs and the reinforcement they may receive from like-minded people in partisan echo chambers can make it difficult for them to break free from their paranoid worldview. In such cases, the role of the therapist may be to provide support and guidance to family members and loved ones, helping them to set appropriate boundaries, communicate effectively, and cope with the challenges of living with someone with PPD or paranoia. By fostering a supportive and understanding environment, therapists can help mitigate the impact of these conditions on both the client and their social circle.

Anger, Disappointment, Shame, and Political Partisanship

While personality disorders and mental health conditions can undoubtedly contribute to extreme political partisanship, it is essential to recognize that people who struggle with excessive anger, disappointment, or shame may also be drawn to hyper-partisan movements, even in the absence of a formal diagnosis. These intense emotional states can cut across a variety of psychological profiles. Still, their common feature is a profound sense of discontent with oneself, others, or the world at large.

Anger, disappointment, and shame are complex emotions that often stem from deep-seated feelings of powerlessness, inadequacy, or injustice (Kelly & Lamia, 2018). When these emotions are left unresolved or unprocessed, they can fester, leading people to seek outlets or explanations for their distress. In the context of politics, hyper-partisan ideologies can provide a seductively straightforward narrative that channels these emotions into a clear target or enemy.

For example, consider the case of John, a middle-aged man who has struggled with feelings of anger and disappointment throughout his life. Despite his best efforts, he has never quite achieved the level of success or recognition he believes he deserves, leaving him with a chronic sense of bitterness and resentment. When he encounters a partisan political movement that speaks to his frustrations and offers a clear target for his anger (e.g., immigrants, the wealthy elite, the "liberal agenda"), he feels a sense of validation and purpose. By aligning himself with this movement, he can externalize his anger and disappointment, directing it toward a perceived enemy rather than confronting the more complex and painful root causes of his emotions (Terjesen & Del Vecchio, 2023).

Similarly, people who struggle with deep-seated shame may be drawn to hyper-partisan movements that offer a sense of moral superiority or righteousness. By adopting an "us versus them" mentality and positioning themselves on the "right" side of a political divide, they can temporarily alleviate their shame and feel a sense of belonging and purpose. However, this relief is often fleeting, as the underlying shame remains unaddressed.

The attraction of hyper-partisan ideologies for people struggling with anger, disappointment, or shame lies in their ability to provide a simplistic yet powerful narrative that offers clear villains, heroes, and solutions. These ideologies often rely on binary thinking, painting the world in stark black-and-white terms that leave little room for subtlety or complexity. For people who are already grappling with intense and painful emotions, this simplicity can be comforting, as it provides a clear target for their distress and a sense of certainty in an uncertain world.

Moreover, hyper-partisan movements often foster an intense sense of community and belonging, which can be particularly appealing to those who feel alienated, marginalized, or misunderstood. By joining a group of like-minded people who share their anger, disappointment, or shame, they can feel validated and supported, even if this support is ultimately based on a shared sense of grievance rather than genuine connection or understanding.

While the allure of hyper-partisan ideologies for people struggling with these emotions is understandable, it is ultimately maladaptive. Externalizing their distress and focusing on perceived enemies or injustices may temporarily alleviate their painful feelings. Still, they do not address the underlying causes of their anger, disappointment, or shame. Instead, they risk becoming further entrenched in a polarized worldview that only perpetuates their emotional distress and alienates them from those who do not share their views.

Treating people who are drawn to hyper-partisan movements due to their problematic emotional experiences requires a compassionate approach that acknowledges the complexity of their situation while also challenging the maladaptive beliefs and behaviors that perpetuate their distress. One key aspect of treatment is helping these people develop greater self-awareness and emotional regulation skills. This may involve teaching mindfulness techniques or classic relaxation training, such as deep breathing or progressive muscle relaxation, to help them better manage their intense emotions in the moment. By learning to observe their anger, disappointment, or shame without becoming overwhelmed by them, they can start to create space for more adaptive coping strategies. Helping clients to understand that they are not their feelings or thoughts, but rather the observer of those phenomena can be useful in allowing them to become more introspective and less reactive. It allows them to create am "observation gap" between feeling provoked and reacting. They can then make conscious choices about how to respond rather than being triggered and reacting.

CBT can also be a valuable tool in helping these clients identify and challenge the distorted thoughts and beliefs that fuel their emotional distress (Dobson, 2024). For example, a therapist using CBT might help John recognize how his all-or-nothing thinking patterns contribute to his chronic sense of disappointment and resentment. By learning to reframe his experiences in a more balanced and realistic way, he can start to develop a realistic understanding of himself and the world around him.

Another crucial aspect of treatment is helping these people explore and process the root causes of their anger, disappointment, or shame. This can also occur in cognitive therapy, though only if attention is paid to the importance of the therapeutic relationship (Wenzel, 2025); a variety of therapies may involve delving into their early life experiences, attachment histories, or experiences of trauma or adversity. By developing a deeper understanding of the origins of their emotional pain, they can start to develop self-compassion and a sense of perspective that allows them to relate to their emotions with more empathy.

Interpersonal and psychodynamic therapies can be particularly useful in this regard, as they focus on exploring the individual's patterns of relating to others and understanding how these patterns may be rooted in early experiences or unresolved emotional conflicts. By developing insight into their relational dynamics and learning to communicate their emotions more adaptively, people can start to build more fulfilling and authentic connections with others.

In our experience, therapists must directly address the individual's involvement in hyper-partisan movements, exploring how their political beliefs and behaviors may reinforce their emotional distress. This requires a delicate balance of validating the individual's experiences and emotions while also challenging the rigid, black-and-white thinking that often characterizes hyper-partisan ideologies.

The goal of treatment for people drawn to hyper-partisan movements due to excessive anger, disappointment, or shame is not to change their fundamental political orientation, rather to help them develop a more flexible and adaptive way of relating to their emotions and the world around them. By building emotional resilience, self-awareness, and interpersonal skills, they can learn to channel their passions more constructively and engage in political discourse from a place of greater wholeness and authenticity.

Bipolar Disorder

Bipolar disorder may mimic personality disorders but it is recognized as a separate condition (Swales et al., 2024). We were very surprised to see clinicians note that bipolar disorder can complicate partisan sentiment. However, this makes sense. Bipolar disorder, characterized by extreme mood swings, including periods of mania or hypomania and depression, can also be misinterpreted in a politically charged environment (Dinerman, Davis, Janos, Walsh, & Sylvia, 2020). During manic or hypomanic episodes, people may display behaviors that resemble the intense passion and conviction of hyper-partisanship. For example, the heightened energy, enthusiasm, and grandiosity seen in manic episodes can mirror the enthusiasm with which some hyper-partisan people express their political views. Rapid speech and flight of ideas, common symptoms of mania, might manifest as quickly jumping from one political topic to another or speaking energetically and somewhat disjointedly, resembling the enthusiasm seen in hyper-partisan debates.

Impulsivity and poor judgment, also associated with manic phases, could lead to bold political statements or actions aligned with extreme activism. A clinician may wonder, "Is this person truly bipolar, or do they simply have very fervent beliefs?" A detailed family history is often helpful to answer this question. However, a history of radical shifts in political or even religious allegiance may provide a clue, although not definitively, to an underlying bipolar disorder.

Bipolar II disorder is characterized by depressive episodes and less severe hypomanic episodes (Dinerman et al., 2020) and is particularly prone to misdiagnosis in a political context. The subtlety of hypomania, often overshadowed by depressive symptoms, can be easily overlooked or misinterpreted as merely good moods or high productivity. Clinicians may attribute the individual's amplified expressions of political opinions during hypomanic episodes to hyper-partisanship, especially if these expressions coincide with the rise of polarizing echo chambers on social media platforms. The case study below illustrates how difficult it can be to detect true bipolar signals from the noise of political activism.

DAMION, A PROGRESSIVE ACTIVIST

Damion, a 32-year-old software engineer, appeared to find deep fulfillment in political activism. With a keen intellect and a passionate heart, he was always at the forefront of progressive causes in his Southern town. When a new issue emerged that aligned with his progressive values, Damion would dive headfirst into activism, organizing events, and mobilizing support through social media. His energy seemed boundless and his enthusiasm infectious.

However, a different side of Damion emerged during the quiet times when there were no pressing political causes. During these periods, he became uncharacteristically sullen, withdrawing from his work and isolating himself at home. His once vibrant social life would come to a halt, replaced by long hours in front of his computer, immersed in coding projects.

Friends noted that his cheerful demeanor would give way to an angry, withdrawn state.

This cyclical pattern of high-energy activism followed by periods of withdrawal puzzled Damion's friends and family. It was not until he sought therapy for what he believed were issues related to burnout and stress, that a deeper understanding of his behavior emerged. During therapy sessions, it became clear that Damion's experiences went beyond the typical fluctuations in mood associated with activism and work stress.

During his high-energy phases, Damion showed signs of hypomania. He had an inflated sense of self-confidence, which often led him to take on numerous tasks simultaneously, believing he could handle them all without difficulty. He talked rapidly, jumped from one political idea to another, and had a reduced need for sleep, sometimes getting by on just a few hours a night. His productivity during these periods was remarkable, but so was his irritability, hypersexuality, and impatience with those who could not keep up with his pace.

Conversely, during his low periods, Damion experienced significant depressive symptoms. He felt an overwhelming sense of hopelessness and fatigue, lost interest in activities he once enjoyed, and struggled with feelings of worthlessness. His ability to concentrate diminished, and he found it challenging to make decisions, even about mundane tasks. These depressive episodes were marked by social withdrawal, a stark contrast to his usual outgoing nature during hypomanic phases.

Upon recognizing these symptoms, Damion's therapist diagnosed him with Bipolar II disorder. This was a turning point in his treatment. Understanding that Damion's mood fluctuations were not merely situational but part of a broader mood disorder allowed for a more effective treatment plan. Damion started on a regimen that included mood stabilizers to help manage his hypomanic and depressive episodes, along with psychotherapy to provide support and strategies for coping with his condition.

With proper treatment, Damion began to notice a significant improvement in his quality of life. He learned to recognize the early signs of his mood swings and developed strategies to manage his energy levels more effectively. While he did not lose his progressive political beliefs, he learned to express them in a less destructive, exhaustive, and extreme manner.

Autism Spectrum Disorder and Partisanship

Autism spectrum disorder (ASD) is a neurodevelopmental condition characterized by challenges in social interaction communication and restricted or repetitive patterns of behavior or interests (Skuse, Greaves-Lord, Rodrigues da Cunha, & Baird, 2024). While ASD is not defined as a personality disorder, it affects most aspects of one's personality. It is not inherently linked to political partisanship, yet some people on the spectrum may exhibit behaviors or thought patterns that resemble those of highly partisan individuals.

Most clinicians now realize that autism is a spectrum disorder, meaning that the severity and manifestation of symptoms can vary widely from person to person (Henderson, Wayland, & White, 2024). Some people with ASD may have significant difficulties with social interaction and communication. In contrast, others may be highly verbal and socially engaged but struggle with more subtle aspects of social reciprocity or understanding, often regarding how to understand and express emotions.

Yet one common misconception about ASD is that people on the spectrum lack empathy.(NO PARAGRAPH BREAK HERE)

In reality, many people with ASD have empathic, compassionate feelings. Still, they may struggle to express or apply them in socially typical ways (Baron-Cohen, 2013). They may have difficulty reading social cues, understanding unspoken social rules, or knowing how to respond appropriately to others' emotions.

Moreover, people with ASD often struggle with theory of mind, or the ability to understand and attribute mental states to others. They may have difficulty recognizing that others have thoughts, beliefs, and perspectives that differ from their own (Baron-Cohen, 2011b). This can make it challenging for them to consider alternative viewpoints or engage in perspective-taking, which is a critical skill in navigating complex political discussions and engaging in anything but solipsistic dialogue.

In the context of political partisanship, people with ASD may be drawn to the clear-cut, black-and-white thinking that often characterizes hyper-partisan ideologies. The social world can be confusing and overwhelming for those on the spectrum, and the simplicity and certainty offered by polarized political narratives may be appealing. They may latch onto a particular ideology or set of beliefs and have difficulty understanding or accepting the validity of opposing perspectives.

Furthermore, the autistic brain is often geared toward pattern recognition and puzzle-solving (Baron-Cohen, 2011a). People with ASD may be drawn to overarching theories or explanations that attempt to make sense of complex social or political phenomena. Once they have identified a pattern or explanation that seems to fit, they may become extremely attached to it and resistant to alternative viewpoints or contradictory evidence.

For example, an individual with ASD may become fixated on a particular conspiracy theory that seems to explain a complex political event or social trend. They may spend countless hours researching and analyzing information related to this theory, becoming increasingly convinced of its validity. When confronted with evidence that contradicts their beliefs, they may become defensive or dismissive, struggling to integrate current information that challenges their established worldview

Therapists need to recognize that people with ASD who exhibit highly partisan behaviors are not necessarily acting out of malice or ill intent. Their rigidity of thought and difficulty with perspective-taking may be rooted in the core features of their neurodevelopmental condition rather than a deliberate choice to be closed-minded or hostile toward others. An example is Tim, below:

TIM

Tim, a 36-year-old computer programmer diagnosed with ASD, exemplifies several core symptoms of the condition. He experiences significant social communication challenges, such as difficulty interpreting social cues and maintaining eye contact, which can impede his ability to engage in face-to-face conversations. Additionally, Tim exhibits repetitive behaviors and a strong preference for routines, often becoming anxious when his daily schedule is disrupted. His deep and intense focus on specific interests, notably politics and technology, further characterizes his ASD, alongside sensory sensitivities that make him prefer quieter, controlled environments.

Tim's intense focus on politics has driven him toward a hyper-partisan stance, predominantly supporting extreme racist causes. This fixation manifests through several distinct behaviors. He filters information, consuming news and content that align exclusively with his political beliefs, thus reinforcing an echo chamber effect where his views are constantly validated. Online, Tim engages in provocative discussions, often trolling individuals with opposing views to provoke reactions, finding a sense of control and satisfaction in these interactions. His cognitive rigidity, a symptom of ASD, contributes to his hyper-partisan stance, making it difficult for him to consider alternative perspectives or the nuances of complex political issues.

The impact of Tim's hyper-partisan behavior on his personal and professional life has been profound. Socially, his provocative online actions have alienated friends and family members with differing political views, leading to increased isolation and a greater reliance on online interactions for social engagement. Professionally, his political beliefs sometimes create tensions with colleagues, affecting his workplace relationships and overall job performance and satisfaction. The constant engagement in online conflicts has also taken an emotional toll on Tim, leading to heightened stress and anxiety.

Despite these challenges, Tim continues to engage in hyper-partisan, racist behavior due to the perceived benefits and sense of control it provides. Online communities that share his political beliefs offer him a sense of belonging and acceptance, a crucial factor given his struggles with face-to-face interactions. These communities provide a platform for him to express his views without the social complexities of offline interactions. However, this reliance on online engagement further entrenches his hyper-partisan stance and exacerbates the difficulties he faces in both his personal and professional life.

One key aspect of treatment for people with ASD who struggle with political partisanship is to help them develop greater social awareness and perspective-taking skills. This may involve explicit instruction in reading social cues, understanding others' emotions, and considering alternative viewpoints. Role-playing exercises, social stories, and video modeling can be helpful tools in this regard.

CBT can also be a valuable approach for people with ASD who exhibit rigid or polarized thinking patterns (Skuse et al., 2024). CBT can help them learn to identify and challenge their automatic thoughts, develop more flexible and adaptive thinking styles, and tolerate uncertainty or ambiguity. By learning to question their assumptions and consider multiple perspectives, they may become more open to engaging in open political discussions.

Another critical aspect of treatment is to help people with ASD find healthy outlets for their interests and passions. As the case of Tim shows, this may involve alternatives to online identities. Many people on the spectrum have intense areas of focus or expertise, which can be channeled in productive ways. Encouraging them to engage in constructive activities related to their particular interests, such as writing, research, or advocacy work, can help them feel more fulfilled and connected to others who share their passions.

Building a solid therapeutic relationship is also essential when collaborating with people with ASD who struggle with political partisanship. Many people on the spectrum have had negative experiences with social rejection or misunderstanding, and they may be initially wary or distrustful of others (Combs, 2024). By creating a safe, nonjudgmental space for them to explore their thoughts and feelings, therapists can help them feel more comfortable opening up and considering new perspectives. It is essential for therapists to be patient and to understand that progress may be slow when collaborating with people with ASD who exhibit highly partisan behaviors. The rigid thinking patterns and social challenges associated with ASD can be deeply entrenched, and it may take time and consistent effort to help them develop greater flexibility and openness to others' viewpoints.

Ultimately, the goal of treatment for people with ASD who struggle with political partisanship is not necessarily to change their political beliefs but rather to help them engage in political discourse in a more adaptive and socially appropriate way. By developing greater social awareness, perspective-taking skills, and flexibility of thought, they can learn to express their views in a way that is respectful of others and open to constructive dialogue.

Consequences of Misdiagnosis

When BPD, bipolar disorder, NPD, HPD, ASPD, PPD, emotional struggles, or ASD are coupled with hyper-partisanship, it can have severe repercussions for the individual and their treatment. Without an accurate diagnosis, clients may not receive the appropriate interventions for their underlying mental health condition, personality disorder, emotional difficulties, or neurodevelopmental differences.

In the case of bipolar disorder, pharmacotherapy is a cornerstone of effective treatment, and its absence can lead to a worsening of symptoms. Similarly, people with BPD, NPD, HPD, ASPD, or PPD may require specific therapeutic approaches that target the core features of their disorders. Those struggling with excessive anger, disappointment, or shame may need help developing emotional regulation skills and processing the root causes of their distress. People with ASD may require support in creating social awareness, perspective-taking abilities, and flexible thinking patterns.

Moreover, being labeled as "hyper-partisan" can carry a stigma that negatively impacts personal relationships and social standing. The individual's behavior, stemming from a mental health condition, emotional struggle, or neurodevelopmental difference, may be met with a lack of understanding and support from their social circle if it is attributed solely to political extremism.

The consequences extend beyond the individual level. On a societal scale, misinterpreting mental health symptoms, emotional distress, or neurodevelopmental differences as political partisanship can contribute to the further polarization and marginalization of those with these challenges. It perpetuates the misconception that these conditions are a matter of personal choice or political ideology rather than legitimate medical or psychological issues requiring support and treatment.

Therapists play a crucial role in navigating the complex intersection of mental health, emotional well-being, neurodevelopmental differences, and political partisanship. They must approach these cases with sensitivity and a deep understanding of the psychological, social, and political factors at play. Psychotherapy that assists individuals in learning more adaptive ways to participate in their political lives is an important resource to help clients become more effective citizens. Political engagement is not a solo endeavor; there's always the need to engage in productive relationships with others and build consensus and coalitions. When psychiatric disorders impede individuals from becoming socially or politically involved in productive ways, psychotherapy can help clients develop cognitive and social skills. Mental health challenges should not be a barrier to full citizenship.

First, therapists must be aware of their own biases and how these may influence their perception of clients. Countertransference, the therapist's emotional response to the client, can be particularly challenging when political beliefs are involved. Therapists must strive to maintain objectivity and avoid projecting their own political views onto their clients.

Secondly, conducting a thorough assessment is essential for accurate diagnosis. Therapists should consider the client's full range of behaviors, emotional patterns, cognitive styles, and personal history rather than focusing solely on their political expressions. Gathering information from multiple sources, including family members and previous healthcare providers, can provide a more comprehensive picture.

Beyond this, therapists must approach these cases with empathy and understanding. Recognizing the complex interplay of mental health, emotional experiences, neurodevelopmental differences, and the sociopolitical context, they should create a safe, nonjudgmental space for clients to explore their thoughts and feelings. The notion that the therapy space is essential for healing is one that is true for even these difficult clients. By fostering open communication and trust, therapists can help clients gain insight into their conditions and develop effective coping strategies.

Therapists should also stay informed about the latest research and best practices in the field. As the understanding of the intersection between mental health, emotional well-being, neurodiversity, and political partisanship evolves, therapists must be prepared to adapt their approaches accordingly. Engaging in continuing education and collaborating with colleagues can help ensure that clients receive the most appropriate and up-to-date care.

Finally, therapists have a role to play in advocating for greater awareness and understanding of mental health conditions, emotional struggles, and neurodevelopmental differences within the broader sociopolitical context. By educating the public, policymakers, and other healthcare professionals about the complexities of these issues, therapists can help reduce stigma, improve access to care, and foster a more compassionate and inclusive society.

Summary

This chapter underscores the intricate relationship between several specific mental health conditions and extreme political partisanship, highlighting the unique challenges therapists face in this context. Through detailed examinations of various personality disorders—such as BPD, bipolar disorder, NPD, HPD, ASPD, and PPD we discuss how traits like rigid thinking, emotional reactivity, and a black-and-white worldview can both manifest in and exacerbate hyper-partisan behavior. It also explores how intense emotions like anger, disappointment, and shame, as well as neurodevelopmental conditions like ASD, can drive individuals toward polarized political movements, further complicating their interpersonal relationships and overall well-being.

References

Babl, A., Gómez Penedo, J. M., Berger, T., Schneider, N., Sachse, R., & Kramer, U. (2022). Change processes in psychotherapy for patients presenting with histrionic personality disorder. *Clinical Psychology & Psychotherapy*. https://doi.org/10.1002/cpp.2769

Baron-Cohen, S. (2011a). The autistic mind: The empathizing-systemizing theory. In E. Hollander, A. Kolevzon, & J. T. Coyle (Eds.), *Textbook of autism spectrum disorders* (pp. 39–47). American Psychiatric Publishing, Inc. https://ulm.idm.oclc.org/login?url=https://search.ebscohost.com/login.aspx?direct=true&db=psyh&AN=2010-23926-003&site=ehost-live

Baron-Cohen, S. (2011b). What is theory of mind, and is it impaired in ASC? In S. Bölte & J. Hallmayer (Eds.), *Autism spectrum conditions: FAQs on autism, Asperger syndrome, and atypical autism answered by international experts* (pp. 136–138).

Hogrefe Publishing. https://ulm.idm.oclc.org/login?url=https://search.ebscohost.com/login.aspx?direct=true&db=psyh&AN=2011-07075-040&site=ehost-live

Baron-Cohen, S. (2013). Empathy deficits in autism and psychopaths: Mirror opposites? In M. R. Banaji & S. A. Gelman (Eds.), *Navigating the social world: What infants, children, and other species can teach us* (pp. 212–215). Oxford University Press. https://doi.org/10.1093/acprof:oso/9780199890712.003.0038

Combs, D. (2024). Supporting neurodivergent and autistic people for their transition into adulthood: Blueprints for education, training, and employment. Routledge. https://doi.org/10.4324/9781003353959

Dinerman, J. G., Davis, B. J., Janos, J. A., Walsh, S. L., & Sylvia, L. G. (2020). Bipolar and related disorders. In A. Chopra, P. Das, & K. Doghramji (Eds.), *Management of sleep disorders in psychiatry* (pp. 304–317). Oxford University Press. https://doi.org/10.1093/med/9780190929671.003.0018

Dobson, K. S. (2024). Cognitive restructuring in the treatment of depression. In Clinical depression: An individualized, biopsychosocial approach to assessment and treatment (pp. 149–166). American Psychological Association. https://doi.org/10.1037/0000398-009

Elleuch, D. (2024). Narcissistic Personality Disorder through psycholinguistic analysis and neuroscientific correlates. Frontiers in Behavioral Neuroscience, *18*. https://doi.org/10.3389/fnbeh.2024.1354258

Hamlat, E. J., Young, J. F., & Hankin, B. L. (2020). Developmental course of personality disorder traits in childhood and adolescence. *Journal of Personality Disorders*, *34*(Suppl B), 25–43. https://doi.org/10.1521/pedi_2019_33_433

Henderson, D., Wayland, S., & White, J. (2024). Is this autism? A companion guide for diagnosing. Routledge. https://doi.org/10.4324/9781003403838

Kapil-Pair, K. N., Landa, Y., Hansen, M. C., Vaccaro, D. H., & Goodman, M. (2021). Psychosis in personality disorders. In C. A. Tamminga, E. I. Ivleva, U. Reininghaus, & J. van Os (Eds.), *Psychotic disorders: Comprehensive conceptualization and treatments* (pp. 59–69). Oxford University Press. https://doi.org/10.1093/med/9780190653279.003.0008

Kelly, V. C., Jr., & Lamia, M. C. (2018). The upside of shame: Therapeutic interventions using the positive aspects of a 'negative' emotion. W. W. Norton & Co. https://ulm.idm.oclc.org/login?url=https://search.ebscohost.com/login.aspx?direct=true&db=psyh&AN=2017-54743-000&site=ehost-live

Kockler, T. D., Santangelo, P. S., Eid, M., Kuehner, C., Bohus, M., Schmaedeke, S., & Ebner-Priemer, U. W. (2022). Self-esteem instability might be more characteristic of borderline personality disorder than affective instability: Findings from an e-diary study with clinical and healthy controls. *Journal of Psychopathology and Clinical Science*, *131*(3), 301–313. https://doi.org/10.1037/abn0000731

Lee, R., & Santos, E. (2022). Paranoid personalities (vigilant style). In R. E. Feinstein (Ed.), *Personality disorders* (pp. 421–439). Oxford University Press. https://ulm.idm.oclc.org/login?url=https://search.ebscohost.com/login.aspx?direct=true&db=psyh&AN=2023-22399-016&site=ehost-live

Magid, M., & Fox, I. (2022). Histrionic personality disorder. In R. E. Feinstein (Ed.), *Personality disorders* (pp. 501–522). Oxford University Press. https://ulm.idm.oclc.org/login?url=https://search.ebscohost.com/login.aspx?direct=true&db=psyh&AN=2023-22399-020&site=ehost-live

Skuse, D., Greaves-Lord, K., Rodrigues da Cunha, G., & Baird, G. (2024). Autism spectrum disorder. In G. M. Reed, P. L. J. Ritchie, A. Maercker, & T. J. Rebello (Eds.), *A psychological approach to diagnosis: Using the ICD-11 as a framework* (pp. 61–77). American Psychological Association. https://doi.org/10.1037/0000392-004

Smith, T. L., & Catanzano, S. M. (2022). Psychopharmacology of personality disorders. In R. E. Feinstein (Ed.), *Personality disorders* (pp. 393–417). Oxford University Press. https://ulm.idm.oclc.org/login?url=https://search.ebscohost.com/login.aspx?direct=true&db=psyh&AN=2023-22399-015&site=ehost-live

Stone, M. H. (2014). Paranoid, schizotypal, and schizoid personality disorders. In G. O. Gabbard (Ed.), *Gabbard's treatments of psychiatric disorders* (5th ed., pp. 999–1014). American Psychiatric Publishing, Inc. https://ulm.idm.oclc.org/login?url=https://search.ebscohost.com/login.aspx?direct=true&db=psyh&AN=2014-23557-068&site=ehost-live

Swales, M. A. (2019). Dialectical behaviour therapy: Development and distinctive features. In M. A. Swales (Ed.), *The Oxford handbook of dialectical behaviour therapy* (pp. 3–19). Oxford University Press. https://ulm.idm.oclc.org/login?url=https://search.ebscohost.com/login.aspx?direct=true&db=psyh&AN=2018-39784-001&site=ehost-live

Swales, M. A., Clark, L. A., & Farnam, A. (2024). Personality disorder. In G. M. Reed, P. L. J. Ritchie, A. Maercker, & T. J. Rebello (Eds.), *A psychological approach to diagnosis: Using the ICD-11 as a framework* (pp. 311–326). American Psychological Association. https://doi.org/10.1037/0000392-017

Terjesen, M. D., & Del Vecchio, T. (2023). Handbook of training and supervision in cognitive behavioral therapy. Springer Nature Switzerland AG. https://doi.org/10.1007/978-3-031-33735-2

Ward, M., Benjamin, I., & Zimmerman, M. (2022). The clinical characteristics of patients with borderline personality disorder in different treatment settings. *Journal of Personality Disorders*, *36*(2), 217–229. https://doi.org/10.1521/pedi_2021_35_536

Wenzel, A. (2025). Therapeutic relationship-focused cognitive behavioral therapy. American Psychological Association. https://doi.org/10.1037/0000424-000

9

POLITICS, SUBSTANCE ABUSE, AND ADDICTIVE BEHAVIORS

Politics and Addictions

Addictive behaviors of all types, including alcohol, nicotine use, stimulants, and opiates, kill more than 700,000 people annually in the United States. This number is more than 13 times the number of people who die from gun violence. Over 110,000 people overdose on narcotics each year. Cigarette smoking is responsible for more than 480,000 deaths per year in the United States, including more than 41,000 deaths resulting from secondhand smoke exposure. This equates to about one in five deaths annually, or 1,300 deaths every day (Centers for Disease Control and Prevention, 2023).

Excessive alcohol use was responsible for more than 140,000 deaths in the United States each year from 2015 to 2019, or more than 380 deaths per day (Centers for Disease Control and Prevention, 2023). The number of people who die from disordered eating, gambling, and other behavioral addictions has not been adequately estimated and is not included in the 22,000 people who take their own lives with substance-related contributing factors (National Institute on Drug Abuse, 2022).

In 2023, about 46.3 million people aged 12 or older (or 16.5% of the population) met the applicable diagnostic criteria for having a substance use disorder. This includes 29.5 million people classified as having an alcohol use disorder and 24 million people classified as having a drug use disorder (Substance Abuse and Mental Health Services Administration, 2023). Alternative estimation methods may render an even higher number (Mojtabai, 2022; Narayanan, Harding, Saba, Conley, & Gordon, 2016).

DOI: 10.4324/9781032651217-9

The data indicates that about one in six people in the United States has a diagnosable substance abuse problem. Despite this staggering number, people across the political spectrum have been unable to unify and successfully address the massive problem of addiction. While there are similarities in concern among both major political parties, there are also substantial disagreements (Narayanan et al., 2016). These disagreements can fragment the development of an evidence-based, humane social policy for preventing and treating addiction. This failure costs many lives and ruins many more. Ideology too often impairs rational discussion and policies in what everyone realizes is a national crisis.

Conservative and liberal ideologies often differ regarding the conceptualization of addiction and its appropriate treatment. Typically, more conservative and traditional approaches prioritize punitive measures and criminalization. At the same time, liberal perspectives often emphasize rehabilitation and public health approaches (Flanagan, 2017). Conservatives tend to see both substance based and other addictions, such as gambling, as a personal choice and beyond societal intervention. In contrast, liberals often focus on several social problems, such as poverty, that are causally related and may advocate for radical societal changes to address this issue (Fraser et al., 2017). This also cuts across social class, with poorer people less likely to hold stigmatizing views of addiction (Miller, Cuthbertson, & Loveridge, 2022).

Stigma regarding addictive behavior is often a complicating factor in treatment (Janet, Hannah, & Stephan, 2020). Political attitudes can shape stigmatization regarding how our society views addiction. There can be a tendency in conservative circles to view addiction as a moral failing or choice, leading to disgrace and shame. Liberal ideologies may be more inclined to view addiction as a disease, emphasizing the need for medical treatment and compassion. This can help reduce stigma and often encourages people to seek therapy, perhaps early in their addiction process. This belief, however, may also reduce personal accountability and possibly induce helplessness regarding choices.

A region or country's ideology can influence attitudes toward addiction. In general, more conservative areas emphasize drug prevention through law enforcement. This policy is, at best, equivocal in its results. Political leanings may also influence how governments allocate addiction-related funding. Liberal governments may spend more public money on health initiatives, including addiction treatment and prevention. The private sector may play a more significant role in more conservative areas. Sometimes, this can lead to more innovative treatment, but often, this results in higher costs and limited access for some populations. As we saw in the 1980s with crack cocaine, political decisions and ideology helped determine which drugs of abuse society saw as essential problems which require a response. Even research and education are influenced by politics. Grant funding may sometimes reflect both ideology and science as the recent history of funding for research on hallucinogens shows.

An example of the influence of ideology is attitudes toward harm reduction approaches, a science-based set of interventions that generally have substantial empirical support. Harm reduction is a philosophy that states some degree of substance use or exposure to an addictive substance will inevitably occur. By reducing the harm and recognizing that prohibition is often futile, it is believed that this will result in a better treatment outcome and less damage to society. They focus on minimizing adverse health outcomes through programs such as needle exchanges or controlled gambling. Politically, more liberal people generally favor harm reduction policies. More conservative people typically tend to prefer abstinence-based approaches, which may ignore the complexities of addiction and may not be effective for everyone.

Ideology can also influence someone's perceived need for treatment and perhaps also their choice of drugs of abuse. There is presently no research showing that ideology is associated with a specific drug of choice or addiction severity. Historically, liberals were more likely to smoke marijuana, while conservatives preferred alcohol. Anecdotal evidence from the 1970s suggested that "straights" (conservatives) drank alcohol, while "hippies" (liberals) smoked marijuana and used hallucinogens (Koran, 1972). Today, this distinction is irrelevant as polydrug abuse occurs across the political spectrum (Labaš, 2016).

Politics as a Stressor for Addictions

F__ it all. I decided I would stay drunk until they elected a decent president. If you can't take that, then F__ you, too.

Politics can be cognitively taxing and stressful, whether one keeps up with it through cable television, social media, or other mediums. Some people say they abuse drugs or alcohol to cope with these stressors. While mental health professionals might initially dismiss these claims as excuses, they seem to be increasing and warrant consideration.

There are many reasons why addictive behaviors can be triggered by stress. Clinical accounts suggest that political events may serve as triggers for substance use or relapse in some people. They may also trigger behavioral addictions, such as excessive gambling or spending. The perception and meaning ascribed to political events can significantly impact stress levels for many people. For some, political events or media accounts can be excessively distressing, encouraging them to turn to alcohol, other drugs, or other addictive experiences for relief. Political tensions in families or relationships can also be triggers for intoxication or relapse.

Alcohol use is particularly problematic in this context. Unlike marijuana or most hallucinogens, alcohol can induce agitation and anger, leading to disinhibited behaviors and destructive interactions. These can range from demeaning comments, such as "Gotcha again, dumb 'libtards'," to more extreme reactions encountered on social media and other platforms. Anecdotal accounts in counseling suggest that spouses or partners often face challenges with alcoholic partners who become "fired up" on social media which triggers drinking or escalates while they are intoxicated. An example is John, below, a Republican married to a very progressive partner who is now in alcohol recovery.

John

I hate to admit it, but I started drinking a bit every night because my wife wouldn't shut up about her stupid woke issues. We'd sit down, watch Netflix, whatever, and she would go on and on. I knew I could be in a bad mood or have a few and I would be fine, real happy, smooth it over. I guess it did not work out well.

Beyond the Political Spectrum: Prioritizing Addiction Recovery Over Ideology

Addiction is a complex issue that affects people from all walks of life, regardless of their political beliefs. However, some people may use their political convictions as reason to avoid seeking help for their addictions. This can be a dangerous and counterproductive approach, as it can prevent people from receiving the support and treatment they need to overcome their addictive behaviors.

One way in which people may use their political beliefs to avoid seeking treatment is by insisting on working with a therapist or counselor who shares their political views. For example, a person who identifies as a liberal may refuse to seek help from a therapist who is known to be conservative, or vice versa. While it is understandable that people may feel more comfortable working with someone who shares their values and beliefs, this approach can be limiting and may prevent them from receiving the best possible care. An example is Scott, a very far right conservative who had refused to find help for his alcohol abuse until threatened with divorce. In his first session with one of the authors, he stated:

I know that therapists are liberals. Friends told me that the whole "addiction industry" is just a way for liberals to try and control what we believe and what we do. I drink to cope with the 'bull shit' that I hear from the liberal press. I wouldn't be here if not for my wife telling me she's leaving unless I stop. She's gotten scared a few times recently when my anger and frustration got a bit over the line while I'm drinking.

People who are behaving compulsively or abusing a substance may be ambivalent about behavior change. Addiction often hijacks not only the pleasure centers of the brain but also reasoning, logic, and motivation. Often, any excuse, however irrational, may help continue the addiction. Consequently, concerns that "*I only can really be understood by a progressive lesbian therapist*" or "*My counselor must be a Catholic Christian Republican*" may have cultural resonance, but these requests often impede focusing on the addictive behavior in a timely fashion. Similarly, a person who is attempting to avoid narcotics and insists that their counselor "*Must have smoked weed*" is also setting up an obstacle, an excuse, otherwise known as resistance. This type of thinking can be dangerous, as it can prevent people from receiving the information, support, and guidance they need to overcome their addiction. It can also reinforce the idea that addiction is a personal choice or part of a lifestyle rather than a medical condition that requires professional treatment.

Another way in which people may use their political beliefs to avoid seeking help for addictions is by dismissing or minimizing the severity of their problem. A person who identifies as a libertarian may argue that their habitual cocaine use is a personal choice and that they have the right to do what they want with their own body. Similarly, a progressive person might justify their heroin habit because they are victims of a racist, misogynistic, oppressive society. One of the authors recently worked with a politically progressive person with marijuana usage that interfered with her life. She downplayed the disruptions and her psychological dependence by saying that in the small town where she lives, all liberals stay high. "*It's how we cope with the Trumpers.*"

Politically active people may also feel pressured to hide their own addictions or the addictions of their family members due to the potential for stigma and negative consequences. In recent years, we have seen examples in the United States where having a family member with an addiction has been used as a political weapon against candidates and elected officials. This vicarious stigma can be incredibly damaging and may prevent people from seeking the help they need out of fear of jeopardizing their political careers or reputations.

Addressing Potential Political Differences Directly

Addiction treatment is a deeply personal and often challenging process that requires a high degree of empathy, understanding, and a nonjudgmental approach from therapists. However, few topics in counseling or psychotherapy are more likely to generate intense political feelings than addiction. Political biases can significantly impact the efficacy of treatment by influencing how therapists perceive and interact with their clients. For instance, a therapist with strong liberal views might unconsciously judge a client who expresses conservative beliefs, or vice versa. This can create an environment where the client feels misunderstood or judged, hindering open communication and trust, which are essential for effective therapy.

Political biases can also affect the therapeutic goals and strategies a therapist employs. A therapist's political beliefs might shape their understanding of the causes of addiction and the best approaches for treatment. A therapist with a conservative outlook might emphasize personal responsibility and self-discipline, while a more liberal therapist might focus on social determinants and systemic factors contributing to addiction. Such divergent perspectives can lead to a mismatch between the therapist's approach and the client's needs or expectations, potentially compromising treatment outcomes.

The susceptibility of addiction treatment to political bias is further complicated by the societal and cultural contexts in which both clients and therapists operate. Political polarization in society can exacerbate these biases, as therapists and clients might bring their own partisan views into the therapy space. This can manifest in subtle ways, such as the language used to describe addiction, the interpretation of client behaviors, or the perceived root causes of their addiction. Discussions around harm reduction strategies, like needle exchange programs or safe injection sites, might be colored by the therapist's political stance, influencing how these strategies are presented to and received by the client.

To address therapist biases in addiction treatment, therapists must commit to self-awareness and ongoing professional development. This involves actively engaging in reflection on their own beliefs and how these might influence their practice. As we have advocated throughout this volume, therapists should seek supervision, participate in bias training, and foster an open, inclusive therapeutic environment where clients feel safe to express their beliefs without fear of judgment. By acknowledging and mitigating their own biases, therapists can provide more effective, empathetic, and personalized care, ultimately improving treatment outcomes for clients struggling with addiction.

In substance abuse treatment, perhaps more than any other treatment, addressing political differences between the therapist and the client *early on* is crucial for establishing a solid therapeutic alliance and ensuring the client's engagement in the recovery process. Building a trusting relationship is important for any successful therapy, but it is a critical factor in working with addicted clients. Ignoring or avoiding these differences can create barriers to effective treatment and hinder the client's progress. By openly discussing political concerns, the therapist demonstrates a willingness to understand and validate the client's perspective, fostering a sense of trust and rapport. A reminder that political discussions in therapy are not undertaken with the goal of changing the client's mind, but with the intention of better understanding the client's values and worldview.

Failing to address political differences, as one of our clients noted, "sweeping them under the rug," can cause clients' feelings to fester and interfere with the therapeutic process. Clients who feel that their beliefs are not respected or understood may become resistant to treatment, questioning the therapist's ability to provide unbiased and effective care. This resistance can manifest in various ways, such as not fully disclosing important information, not adhering to treatment recommendations, expressing excessive anger, or prematurely terminating therapy. For people experiencing addiction, so much of their lives become secretive and unspoken. The "elephant in the room" is a common experience of avoidance for addicts and their families and friends. As a client of one of the authors expressed, *"I've spent so many years not talking about what's happening to me or paying attention to how I affect others. The last thing I need is more secrets, either mine or yours."* Honesty on the part of the client and therapist is fundamental to addiction recovery. By proactively addressing political differences when working with addicted clients, therapists can mitigate these risks and create a more collaborative and productive therapeutic environment.

Furthermore, addressing political differences early in therapy provides an opportunity to emphasize the nonpartisan nature of substance abuse and the importance of focusing on recovery. Therapists can help clients understand that their political beliefs, while important, should not be a barrier to seeking and receiving the care they need. By framing substance abuse as a universal issue that transcends political affiliations, therapists can help clients shift their focus from political concerns to their overall health, personal growth, life satisfaction, and well-being. This shift in perspective can be empowering for clients, as they learn to prioritize their recovery and develop a stronger sense of self separate from their political identity. The case study, Samantha, is an example of this.

Samantha

Samantha, a 38-year-old politically conservative woman, was referred to treatment for polysubstance abuse, including opioids, stimulants, alcohol, and hallucinogens. She has a history of sexual abuse and domestic violence victimization. During the intake session, Samantha expressed her reluctance to work with the therapist, stating that she would prefer a more conservative therapist who aligns with her political views. She identified herself on social media as a member of an extremist group. She questioned the therapist's ability to provide effective treatment due to perceived political differences. She noted on her intake form that "liberals and communists" were sources of her current problem and "a good day is when I don't have to interact with them."

In the initial sessions with her therapist, who was politically moderate, Samantha was highly guarded and resistant to treatment. She frequently brought up her political beliefs and affiliation with the extremist group, expressing concern that differing political views would hinder her progress in therapy. In fact, in a seeming throwback to the 1950s, she referred to her therapist as a "commie".

Recognizing the importance of addressing Samantha's concerns while also emphasizing the priority of her substance abuse treatment and mental health, the therapist initiated a conversation about the role of political beliefs in therapy. He acknowledged and validated her feelings, emphasizing that it is common for clients to seek a therapist with similar values and experiences. However, he also highlighted the fact that effective therapy relies on evidence-based practices, empathy, and the therapeutic relationship, rather than shared political views.

He further explained that substance abuse and trauma are nonpartisan issues that affect individuals from all walks of life and political backgrounds. He did not try to deny his own political sentiments. He just emphasized that the shared goal was to work together to address Samantha's polysubstance abuse, sexual abuse history, and experiences of domestic violence, regardless of any political differences.

Throughout the sessions, the therapist consistently demonstrated empathy, active listening, and a nonjudgmental attitude. He created a safe and supportive environment where Samantha felt comfortable discussing her struggles and experiences without fear of political judgment. As the therapeutic relationship strengthened, Samantha began to focus more on her recovery and processing her traumas, and less on our political differences.

Samantha eventually recognized that her initial reluctance to work with a therapist with different political views had been a self-imposed barrier to seeking help. She expressed gratitude for the support and guidance she received in therapy and eventually achieved abstinence from addictive substances.

Recovery and Partisan Sentiments

Political views can sometimes change in clients as their recovery process unfolds. This maybe be due to the biases that addiction counselors hold and the direction in which they attempt to influence their clients. We are aware of politically conservative addiction counselors who believe that "genuine" recovery involves becoming more politically aware and right-wing. We are also mindful of more left-leaning people who believe that "true" recovery consists of an awareness of social problems or taking a more progressive stance. Because the experience of recovery can be so life-changing, the process can involve a change in political beliefs irrespective of the political views of the counselor or other helping professional. Usually, these views result in more moderate, thoughtful attitudes and behaviors for the client. As clients think and feel more, they can avoid the stereotypic responses that are often associated with both ideological excesses and addictive behavior patterns such as blaming others for their actions.

Partisan sentiments may not change, but people often become more civil and pleasant in interaction with others who hold different beliefs. One very conservative client stated:

> When I was doing coke (cocaine), I was an arrogant jerk. I thought my God-given task was to humiliate liberals. I haven't changed my politics, but I am not the sarcastic asshole I used to be, at least not as much!

Recovery can also move people in the other direction regarding political polarization. It is not surprising if a person recovering from addiction starts to be interested in political extremism, similar to the way in which they might embrace religious extremism or conspiracy theories. They often look for quick fixes or magical thinking, partly because this may be their propensity. They may also do this partly because they wish to make up for lost time. Recovery from addiction is a scary, uncertain road that may involve profound grief and a sense of lost opportunities and missed years. Finding a higher purpose, even in politics, may be a transitional strategy for preserving dignity, hope, and meaning.

When people reduce or change their addictive behaviors, it affects those around them. We often highlight the positive: better interactions with friends, more work productivity, and most of all, a renewed connection with family members. Yet for families, there is often a more complex process of reintegrating the addicted person into the family. Addictive behaviors often act as distractions from underlying tension, conflict, or other family problems, shifting the focus to dealing with the addiction and avoiding deeper issues. For example, a couple with sexual incompatibility may use heavy drinking as an excuse for minimal intimacy, accepting this dynamic while avoiding the topic.

Having an "identified patient" with an addiction can give other family members a sense of purpose by trying to control, manage, or fix the addicted person. This dynamic allows family members to feel needed and avoid addressing their own issues. Codependency, a pattern of behaviors or thoughts centered around an excessive reliance on another person, often involves focusing on someone else's needs at the expense of one's own. For a codependent family, the addictive behavior, though unhealthy, provides predictable roles and patterns, creating a sense of equilibrium. People adjust to addicted family members and must redefine their roles as the addicted person changes. Family members may feel shame or anger that they are struggling with accepting the personality and new roles a recovering person assumes in the family.

Shelia, a spouse in a same-sex marriage, expressed this eloquently in a family session.

> When my wife was high, I knew I could count on her to be sweet but pretty worthless. The kids and I made excuses for her, but at least there was some predictability. Now that she's sober, it's a bit uncomfortable because we've all had to adjust to the way she wants things done.

Political extremism can also serve a similar function within a family system. For instance, a family may coalesce around a member's outrageous political statements, overlooking other issues like excessive drinking. Similarly, a couple may become overly involved in a political cause, leading their children to disengage and turn to substance abuse or escapism. In these cases, the focus on political extremism helps maintain the family's equilibrium by distracting from other problems and providing a shared focus or purpose, even if it is ultimately unhealthy.

Fernando, a college-age young man, described how political extremism can stabilize a family while simultaneously doing damage.

Fernando

> When my dad (a divorced father of three) was into "Q" (a right-wing conspiracy) and all of that, we knew he had his attention focused somewhere else. He didn't annoy us. He just talked crazy talk, mostly on social media. But he didn't interact with us. My brothers and me, we picked up the slack, kind of. We sort of raised ourselves because we had to. When he stopped with all of that, it was really hard for my brothers, who felt someone who abandoned us was coming back to try to rule over us. I mean, it was tense for a while, and a lot of doors slammed, cursing, and stuff like that. It's still not quite right because we learned to get along without him. I mean, we had to.

The concept of family as a system is more than metaphoric. Treating addiction often requires disrupting long-established roles and patterns, which can initially destabilize the family as new ways of relating emerge. Family members may need to understand that even if the addicted person stays sober, their relationship will not improve if they continue to engage in codependent behaviors. Removing the symptom (addiction and/or political extremism) can result in a temporary deterioration of other areas of functioning, requiring information, support, and guidance for the family to find a new, healthier equilibrium. Near the end of couple's treatment with a woman recovering from alcoholism and her husband, she made the request that "*He needs to stop trying to take a sniff to see if there's alcohol on my breath every time we kiss. I've been sober for two years and it's pissing me off.*"

Addiction can be conceptualized as a complex, nonlinear system with a "gravitational pull" toward repeating the addictive behavior. The progression of addiction is sensitive to initial conditions and can follow unpredictable, nonlinear trajectories over time. Chaotic systems like addiction are susceptible to heightened sensitivity to external stimuli, which can trigger relapse or addictive behavior. These relapses can involve family members or family roles. This is perhaps why many addiction professionals recognize that a systemic orientation is often valuable.

Motivational Interviewing and Value-Aligned Counseling

At one time, practitioners working with addiction issues were likely to use shame as a major motivating force. Most recognize now that avoiding shame in addiction treatment is crucial for several reasons. Shame often leads individuals to feel fundamentally flawed or unworthy, which can significantly undermine their self-worth and motivation to change. This negative self-perception can be a significant barrier to recovery, as it diminishes the belief in one's ability to achieve and maintain sobriety. Moreover, shame triggers defensive behaviors such as withdrawal, secrecy, and aggression, which can interfere with the therapeutic process and hinder open communication and trust between the patient and therapist. These behaviors make it more difficult for individuals to seek help or to be honest about their progress and setbacks during treatment.

Additionally, shame increases stress, anxiety, and depression, exacerbating addictive patterns as individuals may turn to substance use to cope with these painful emotions. Research (Sawyer, Davis, & Gleeson, 2019) has shown that shame is linked to a higher likelihood of relapse because the negative emotions and stress associated with it can trigger cravings and make maintaining sobriety more challenging. Shame also impedes the development of healthy coping mechanisms and emotional regulation skills by keeping individuals stuck in negative thought patterns and behaviors. Furthermore, shame can damage interpersonal relationships, which are often crucial support systems during recovery, leading to isolation and make it harder for individuals to seek and receive support from loved ones.

Motivational interviewing (MI) in counseling represents a significant shift away from shame-based approaches, focusing instead on empathy, collaboration, and respect for the individual's autonomy (Miller & Rollnick, 2013). This technique emphasizes creating a nonjudgmental, supportive environment where clients feel understood and valued. Instead of confronting individuals with their shortcomings, MI encourages them to explore their motivations for change, helping them to identify and articulate their reasons for wanting to overcome addictive patterns. This approach reduces defensiveness and resistance, fostering a more open and honest dialogue between the client and counselor. By validating the client's experiences and feelings, MI builds a trusting relationship that enhances the effectiveness of the therapeutic process.

MI empowers clients by emphasizing their ability to make choices and take control of their recovery journey. This empowerment contrasts sharply with shame-based approaches, which often leave individuals feeling powerless and demoralized. MI techniques such as reflective listening, affirmations, and the elicitation of change talk help clients recognize their strengths and build self-efficacy. By focusing on clients' intrinsic motivations and fostering a sense of self-empowerment, MI supports sustainable change and long-term recovery. This supportive and positive client-centered approach not only promotes lasting behavioral changes but also enhances overall well-being and self-esteem, making it a more effective and humane alternative to shame-based methods.

MI can be enhanced with politically partisan people through Value-Aligned Counseling (VAC) (Russo-Netzer & Atad, 2024). This is a therapeutic approach that directly integrates a client's political beliefs and core values into the treatment process for addiction. By aligning the counseling strategies with a person's sincerely held political orientation, VAC aims to create a more relatable and motivating framework for recovery. This approach recognizes and respects the client's worldview, using it as a foundation to encourage self-reflection, empower personal agency, and promote sustainable change. VAC shares similarities with MI but goes beyond MI by explicitly addressing the deeply held beliefs and values of highly partisan clients.

Both VAC and MI focus on creating a supportive, nonjudgmental environment where clients feel understood and valued, emphasizing collaboration, empathy, and respect for the client's autonomy. Like MI, VAC is centered around the client, prioritizing their perspectives and experiences. It aims to empower clients by helping them explore their motivations and develop intrinsic reasons for change. Both approaches avoid confrontational or shame-based tactics, using reflective listening and affirmations to validate clients' feelings, thereby reducing defensiveness and fostering open communication. Additionally, MI and VAC both emphasize the client's ability to make their own choices and take control of their recovery journey, which is crucial in building self-efficacy and promoting sustainable change.

VAC goes a step further by explicitly incorporating the client's political beliefs and core values into the counseling process. For highly partisan clients, these beliefs are often central to their identity and worldview. By aligning the therapeutic conversation with these values, VAC makes the counseling process more relatable and motivating. The case of Jasmine is an example.

Jasmine

Jasmine is a 33-year-old self-identified conservative and "lapsed Born Again Christian", She explains that she is politically conservative but suffers from extremely heavy weekend drinking and occasional gambling binges. She has tried to return to her Pentecostal church on several occasions but felt too ashamed to maintain that connection. She had several different counselors and therapists but never managed to achieve more than a few weeks without a return to weekend drinking bouts, which usually occur alone. In a series of sessions with Jasmine, her psychologist, Megan, began by establishing a supportive and nonjudgmental environment, emphasizing that they are working together towards Jasmine's goals. Megan starts by exploring Jasmine's core values, particularly focusing on her conservative beliefs in free will, traditional values, and the importance of community and family cohesion.

"Let's talk about some of the values that are important to you," Megan said. It became very clear that the role of independence, autonomy, and a "live free or die" mentality was a cardinal value of Jasmine's.

Megan formulated a successful intervention with this information. "I know that free choice and people not telling you what to do is important. But how do you feel your drinking affects your ability to exercise that free will?" By framing the conversation in this way, Megan invites Jasmine to reflect on how her substance abuse might be limiting her autonomy and ability to make choices aligned with her values. Megan uses this approach to connect with Jasmine's preference for individual liberties within the bounds of her traditional values.

Later, Megan addressed Jasmine's desire for adherence to traditional values. "You mentioned that you hold traditional values in high regard. Can you share more about what those values are and how they guide your life? Do you feel that your drinking conflicts with those values? Is it something your grandparents would do?" This helped Jasmine identify the dissonance between her behaviors and her core beliefs without feeling judged or shamed, leveraging her conservative inclination toward traditional morality and to her family heritage.

In a later session Megan discussed the importance of family and community. "You've spoken about how important your family and community are to you. How do you think your drinking affects those relationships?" By connecting Jasmine's alcohol abuse to potential harm to her valued relationships, Megan encouraged her to consider the broader implications of her actions, acknowledging her conservative view of society as a static entity that enforces morality and limits human excesses.

Megan even addressed Jasmine's distrust of larger institutions by suggesting that alcohol might be more dangerous than people in corporations and government might want her to believe. "Sometimes, the risks of alcohol use are downplayed. You mentioned that you are worried about vaccines and the things in them. I am wondering how you feel about beer? Who knows what the government allows into a can of beer these days? And who really knows how much is safe to drink? This tapped into Jasmine's distrust of big government and preference for small, local governance, a sentiment common among conservatives.

Megan also realized that conservatives may have more harm avoidance and disgust sensitivity. She did not want to evoke shame or guilt, so she was careful in the way she introduced these topics. "I don't drink because it made me anxious the next day. I don't know if it does with you, but when you quit drinking, you will feel a lot less worried about things. That is everyone's experience."

She also used conservatives' proclivity to disgust sensitivity to suggest a more positive daily experience. Laughingly, in a kind way, she noted "Your makeup must look awful after you spend the night drinking! Gosh, next time you drink, take a selfie. I want to see what you look like in the morning." Jasmine laughed and said this was something she thought a lot about and that she could write a country song based on how bad she looked in the mirror after a night of excess. "That's one big reason I want to quit. I'm also getting fat and breaking my nails."

Finally, in a later session, Megan interpreted Jasmine's drinking as a reaction to modern stresses and a longing to return to simpler times. "It sounds like part of your struggle with alcohol might be a response to the stresses of modern life. Maybe you want the good old days when things were simpler. How do you feel about this perspective?" This allows Jasmine to reflect on her motivations and the underlying causes of her substance use.

Throughout their sessions, Megan used reflective listening and affirmations to validate Jasmine's feelings and experiences. For example, "It sounds like you really value your freedom and your ability to live according to your principles. It's understandable that you feel conflicted when drinking and gambling undermine those values." By focusing on Jasmine's intrinsic motivations and aligning the conversation with her values, Megan aims to empower her to recognize the need for change and to take active steps towards recovery.

For highly partisan clients like Jasmine, VAC is particularly important because it respects and incorporates their deeply held beliefs into the therapeutic process. This alignment with their values not only fosters a stronger therapeutic alliance but also enhances the client's motivation and engagement in treatment.

By recognizing and validating their worldview, VAC helps clients navigate their addiction in a manner that feels consistent with their identity, ultimately supporting more effective and lasting recovery.

Self-Help and Social Support in Addiction Treatment

In most cases, even a very partisan person will benefit from referral to a self-help group. While these groups are not for everyone, they work outstandingly well for many people, and it is impossible to predict for whom they will be helpful. Individuals coming into recovery have often been isolated and alienated from family and friends. Recovery means moving out of the relationship with an addictive substance or activity and finding a new community. In his Ted Talk on YouTube titled "Everything You Know About Addiction is Wrong" (July 9, 2015) (https://youtu.be/PY9DcIMGxMs), Johann Hari states that "The opposite of addiction is not sobriety, the opposite of addiction is connection." Finding a supportive group of others who can provide a safe place to be honest and connect to people who are familiar with addiction and recovery is crucial part of maintaining sobriety for many people.

Most self-help groups strive to be nonpartisan. Particularly in more suburban or urban areas there are a variety of meetings for specific populations and visiting several different meetings might be helpful in finding a good fit. They might prefer a religiously or spiritually centered 12-step group combining faith-based approaches or find a group that meets in an area of their community that tends to have more conservative or liberal residents. There are also 12-step groups that are designated for men or women, for LGBTQ+, and for adolescents. Many areas where there are non-English speaking communities offer groups in other languages or meetings based on traditional healing principles for Native Americans and other cultures.

The 12 Steps have a tradition of providing "alternative" versions of the 12 Steps that are more acceptable to agnostics and atheists. The Higher Power and God that are referenced in the 12 Steps can be the human spirit or a belief that people can help each other; it does not need to be a deity. While some people find AA to be "too spiritual," it is difficult to determine whether that is simply treatment reluctance. As one gambler and alcoholic said:

> I don't go for the God talk in AA. To me, it is like a side effect of the treatment. I wouldn't say I like it. But I don't like the side effects of my cancer treatment, either. I take the treatment to stay alive. I am not about to squabble over something petty if most of it works for me.

On the other hand, some people see groups like AA as too conservative, theistic, and lacking in a science base (Glassman, Moensted, Rhodes, & Buus, 2022).

Although they are not as widely available as A.A./N.A., other resources such as "Rational Recovery" which is based on cognitive/rational therapy approaches (Trimpey, 1996) or "Celebrate Recovery" (celebraterecovery.com) which is founded in Christian beliefs and traditions, offer some alternative for finding a support network. There are variations of the 12 Steps for Buddhists as well (Buddhist Recovery Network, n.d.). People who live in rural or isolated areas may not be able to find a group they can attend, but many recovering communities also offer virtual meetings on-line. These are also good alternatives for people who may be too ill to attend live meetings, who don't have reliable transportation, or whose work schedule doesn't fit with meeting times in their areas. The important thing is building a sense of belonging and connection with others who are pursuing the same goal of recovery.

Summary

In this chapter, we have provided an overview of the interface between substance abuse and addictive disorders with partisan politics. Political policies play a role in how we view addictive disorders and what type of programs and assistance we offer those who suffer with addiction. The stress of our contentious political atmosphere and how it impacts people struggling with addiction and their relationships was examined. For mental health professionals working with addiction recovery, several important approaches such as MI and VAC are important clinical approaches that emphasize self-determination and respect in recovery. Finding supportive resources, such as A.A is also encouraged. By understanding the role of politics in addiction and fostering a supportive, nonjudgmental therapeutic environment, mental health professionals can help clients overcome the challenges of addiction and achieve lasting recovery.

References

Buddhist Recovery Network. (n.d.). buddhistrecovery.org/meetings/

Celebrate Recovery. (n.d.). celebraterecovery.com

Centers for Disease Control and Prevention. (2023). *Smoking & tobacco use: Fast facts.* Centers for Disease Control and Prevention.

Flanagan, O. (2017). Willing addicts? Drinkers, dandies, druggies, and other Dionysians. In N. Heather & G. Segal (Eds.), *Addiction and choice: Rethinking the relationship* (pp. 66–81). New York, NY: Oxford University Press.

Fraser, S., Pienaar, K., Dilkes-Frayne, E., Moore, D., Kokanovic, R., Treloar, C., & Dunlop, A. (2017). Addiction stigma and the biopolitics of liberal modernity: A qualitative analysis. *International Journal of Drug Policy, 44*, 192–201. https://doi.org/10.1016/j.drugpo.2017.02.005

Glassman, H. S., Moensted, M., Rhodes, P., & Buus, N. (2022). The politics of belonging in Alcoholics Anonymous: A qualitative interview study. *American Journal of Community Psychology, 70*(1–2), 33–44. https://doi.org/10.1002/ajcp.12568

Hari, J. (2015, July 9). *Everything you know about addiction is wrong.* Ted Talks: You Tube. https://youtu.be/PY9DcIMGxMs

Janet, Z., Hannah, A., & Stephan, A. (2020). Stigma: How it affects the substance use disorder patient [article]. *Substance Abuse Treatment, Prevention, and Policy, 15*(1), 1–4. https://doi.org/10.1186/s13011-020-00288-0

Koran, L. M. (1972). American responses to heroin addiction and marihuana use. In *Social change and human behavior: Mental health challenges of the seventies. DHEW No. (HSM) 72-9122.* US Government Printing Office.

Labaš, S. D. (2016). Alcohol use: Social aspect, gender differences and stigmatization. *Alcoholism and Psychiatry Research, Journal on Psychiatric Research and Addictions, 52*(1), 51–64.

Miller, P. K., Cuthbertson, C. A., & Loveridge, S. (2022). Social status influence on stigma towards mental illness and substance use disorder in the United States. *Community Mental Health Journal, 58*(2), 249–260. https://doi.org/10.1007/s10597-021-00817-6

Miller, W., & Rollnick, S. (2013). *Motivational interviewing: Helping people change* (3rd ed.). New York, NY: Guilford Press.

Mojtabai, R. (2022). Estimating the prevalence of substance use disorders in the US using the benchmark multiplier method. *JAMA Psychiatry, 79*(11), 1074–1080. https://doi.org/10.1001/jamapsychiatry.2022.2756

Narayanan, A. K., Harding, J. D., Jr., Saba, S. K., Conley, J., & Gordon, A. J. (2016). Left, right, and meeting in the middle: Addressing addiction is something we can agree about. *Substance Abuse, 37*(4), 495–497. https://doi.org/10.1080/08897077.2016.1238655

National Institute on Drug Abuse. (2022). *Substance Use in America: Trends and Statistics.* www.samhsa.gov/newsroom/press-announcements/20231113/hhs-samhsa-release-2022-nsduh-data#:~:text=In%202022%2C%2048.7%20million%20people,an%20AUD%20and%20a%20DUD

Russo-Netzer, P. & Atad, O. I. (2024, April 01). Activating values intervention: An integrative pathway to well-being. *Frontiers Psychology, 15.* https://doi.org/10.3389/fpsyg.2024

Sawyer, F., Davis, P., & Gleeson, K. (2019). Is shame a barrier to sobriety? A narrative analysis of those in recovery. *Drugs: Education, Prevention and Policy, 27*(1), 79–85. https://doi.org/10.1080/09687637.2019.1572071

Substance Abuse and Mental Health Services Administration (SAMHSA). (2023). *Mental health and substance abuse disorders.* www.samhsa.gov/find-help/disorder

Trimpey, J. (1996). *Rational recovery: The new cure for substance addiction.* New York, NY: Gallery Books.

10

WORKING WITH POLARIZATION IN RELATIONSHIPS AND FAMILIES

The Beginning of Relationships: To Date or Not to Date?

Some mental health professionals may not be aware, but politics has entered the dating world. Relationship therapists report more clients than ever who are concerned that they meet someone to date who shares their political values. Western dating practices prioritize emotional connection and intimacy. Couples typically seek partners who share their values, interests, and emotional needs, fostering deeper bonds beyond physical attraction. Finding a compatible partner has always been challenging. Historically, a potential partner's ancestry, financial status, religion, education level, shared interests, social status, and other factors have been significant in deciding whether to date someone. Now, political affiliation often serves as a preferred, quick metric for evaluating someone's values and world views.

For many, knowing someone's political orientation provides insight into their world view, and becomes a make-or-break factor in deciding whether to pursue a relationship. Political positions have come to signify someone's core beliefs and perspectives on social and ideological issues. People on both the left and right often view anyone who disagrees with them as simply uninformed, misguided, or downright immoral rather than having legitimate differences of opinion. This tendency to vilify those with opposing views can extend to dating choices, where sharing partisan alignment signals compatibility on all sorts of social and moral positions.

Western relationship models are also becoming increasingly diverse and fluid. There's no one-size-fits-all approach. Some couples choose cohabitation without marriage, while others prioritize emotional intimacy over physical

DOI: 10.4324/9781032651217-10

intimacy. Online dating platforms and social media have dramatically transformed courtship for many people. Internet dating provides avenues for meeting people, filtering preferences, and facilitating communication. However, these tools also present challenges like unrealistic expectations and potential for shallow connections which can be complicated by concerns over political orientations. Other couples choose various degrees of commitment, such as open relationships, or sexual and gender orientations that were previously not as widely acceptable or available. For example, "hookup culture" can lead to casual intimacy without commitment. Essentially, online dating resources offer connections for everything from monogamous, non-sexual relationships to multiple partner combinations or "swinging."

Navigating these complexities requires clear communication, self-awareness, and emotional intelligence. All of these may be impaired when people are also negotiating strong feelings regarding the partisan differences of their potential partner and are worried regarding how these sentiments may play out in their relationship over time. The most common question is "What would I have in common with someone from the other side of the political divide?"

Recent surveys indicate a significant ideological divide between young men and women, complicating dating prospects. In 2021, 44% of women identified as liberal, while only 25% of men did. A decade ago, the difference was much smaller, with 30% of women and 27% of men identifying as liberal (Survey Center on American Life, 2022). This growing divide makes it increasingly unlikely for individuals to consider dating someone with opposing political views, as political compatibility has become a crucial aspect of finding a life partner. Some dating websites now allow participants to overtly filter or exclude prospective partners based on expressed liberal or conservative leanings. Yet finding a romantic match in a time of extreme political rancor may still prove challenging.

Surveys conducted by Match.com (2020) and Change Research (2023) reveal that a significant percentage of singles prioritize political compatibility in dating. The Change Research survey showed that 76% of women would not date someone who supported Trump, while 64% of men would not date someone they perceived as a "communist." This emphasis on political alignment reflects the deepening polarization in society and its impact on personal relationships.

To help navigate these complexities, counselors should foster open communication and promote self-awareness among clients. Encouraging early discussions about political views can help identify potential deal-breakers and reduce future conflicts. Teaching effective communication skills, emphasizing empathy, active listening, and non-defensive communication, can facilitate respectful discussions about political differences. Additionally, helping clients identify their core values and reflect on what aspects of a partner's political views are non-negotiable can aid in making informed decisions about relationships.

This approach ensures that clients enter relationships with a clear understanding of their priorities and boundaries.

Balancing political and personal compatibility is also essential for maintaining healthy relationships. Counselors and therapists should help clients focus on shared interests and values beyond politics to foster connection and common ground. Promoting emotional intelligence can enable clients to navigate political disagreements with sensitivity and understanding, reducing the potential for conflict. Additionally, challenging stereotypes and fostering tolerance can help clients view individuals as multifaceted rather than reducing them to their political affiliations, promoting greater acceptance of differing viewpoints. This balanced approach can enrich relationships and lead to personal growth.

Using online platforms mindfully is another important aspect of relationship counseling that mental health professionals might address. Educating clients on the benefits and pitfalls of using online dating platforms that filter based on political preferences can help manage expectations and encourage realistic approaches to finding compatible partners. Encouraging authenticity in online profiles, including political views, can attract like-minded partners and reduce the likelihood of future conflicts. Understanding the dynamics of online dating and the potential for shallow, single-issue based connections can help clients approach these platforms with a balanced perspective, seeking genuine compatibility beyond political alignment.

United We Stand, Divided We Fall: The Role of Political Similarity in Longer Term Compatibility

Once couples do connect, political similarity can play an essential role in relationship satisfaction. Studies indicate that couples with similar political views report greater satisfaction and are more likely to engage in political activities together (Peacock & Pederson, 2022). The shared values and beliefs that come with political alignment provide a foundation for mutual respect and understanding, crucial elements for a successful relationship. Shared political orientations support greater long-term couple satisfaction. Peacock and Pederson (2022) also found that political similarity correlated with higher relationship fulfillment and engagement in the partnership. Shared political values facilitate agreements on parenting approaches, social issues, and family decision-making. They also enable more constructive forms of communication emphasized by leading couple therapists, including engaged listening, validating partners' perspectives, and maintaining positivity (Gottman & Silver, 2015; Sauerheber et al., 2021). Without significant partisan differences, there are fewer triggers for contempt, criticism, and other destructive communication patterns.

How partners express their political views significantly affects relationship dynamics. Constructive discussions, engagement, humor, and maintaining positivity are crucial for marital satisfaction, especially when there are significant differences in values and worldviews. Couples who communicate openly and respectfully about their political beliefs are more likely to navigate these differences without damaging their relationship. Mutual respect is the foundation for success.

Psychoanalyst Orna Guralnik sees political debates permeating couple conflict around power, privilege, gender norms, and other social issues (Guralnik, 2023). Partners can frequently view each other's political opinions as irrational or immoral. Guralnik notes, one of the most difficult challenges for couples is getting them to see beyond their entrenched perspectives of perceived radical "otherness" in their partner. Successfully bridging political divides rests on valuing the relationship above partisan loyalties, avoiding moral condemnation, and accepting legitimate disagreements between caring partners.

Discussion expressiveness and frequency appear to exert the most influence on how connected we feel to each other regarding political beliefs. Maintenance behaviors, such as engagement instead of withdrawal and a general positivity toward their partner and relationship, are positively correlated with marital satisfaction (Sauerheber et al., 2021; Gottman & Silver, 2015). These types of interactions are more likely to be seen in relationships where significant differences in values and world views are minimized. Indeed, political similarity in a couple reduces the possibility of arguments about how we assess and react to issues that are entwined in political debates, like immigration and climate change.

Jeanne Safer, a psychoanalyst with over 45 years of experience, explores how couples can stay connected despite their divergent political beliefs in the aptly titled book, "*I Love You, but I Hate Your Politics: How to Protect Your Intimate Relationships in a Poisonous Partisan World*" (2019). She relates her experiences with couples in her practice and with her own marriage of several decades to a husband who is her political opposite. She is a liberal, married for almost 40 years to a conservative. For the book, she interviewed 50 individuals and couples who were trying to find their way out of constant political bickering. Safer believes that "Nobody has to settle for political misery at home. With effort, self-awareness, and tact, many bipartisan couples really do figure out how to revere each other despite serious differences of opinion" (Safer, 2019, pp. 125–126).

Safer (2019) suggests several strategies for couples to bridge the political chasm. These include prioritizing love over politics, avoiding attempts to convert each other, and engaging in respectful, open-minded discussions. She emphasizes the importance of focusing on each other's positive traits and maintaining a spirit of goodwill and respect. Couples who acknowledge the belief that "I love my spouse more than I love my country" can prioritize their love for each other. These couples avoid trying to convert each other politically, appreciating each other's character over opinions, and listening more than talking. Keeping a respectful, calm tone and assuming good faith in their partner are also important. Lowering defensiveness by focusing on values rather than issues, and engaging in good-natured political disputes without holding grudges, can help couples navigate political differences.

Seeing our partner in the full context of who they are is the priority; a good parent, a valued companion, someone who's funny, considerate, reliable, kind. It's important to broaden how we assess who our partner is in a more balanced and complete way. Partners let go of the desire to change each other's mind about politics so that they can offer acceptance and even appreciation. We don't have to agree but can learn to love beyond our differences.

Parent/Child Divides

"Till Death Us Do Part" is a notable British television sitcom that aired from 1965 to 1975. The show, which had spinoffs for the next 23 years, centered on the contentious relationship between a conservative family patriarch Alf and his liberal son-in-law, Mikes. The recurrent theme reflected and satirized the social and political tensions of the time confronting racism, sexism, and class conflict. "Till Death Us Do Part" significantly influenced television producer Norman Lear's highly rated show "All in the Family" in the United States, which adapted its core premise and characters to American settings and audiences. This format further inspired a wave of similar sitcoms worldwide, including "Sons and Daughters" in Australia, "Ein Herz und eine Seele" in Germany, and "Mitico Alfredo" in Italy. These shows not only entertained but also encouraged viewers to confront and reflect on their own prejudices and societal issues.

Shows like these highlighted the importance of maintaining respectful relationships despite profound disagreements among family members. These shows humorously provided a template for handling political and ideological differences within families, demonstrating that it is possible to engage in heated debates while maintaining familial bonds. The issues discussed were very controversial, but the way they were addressed was "sensitively contentious." There was not an expectation of agreement so much as an "agree to disagree" approach to political discussions. Issues had to be discussed honestly and perhaps harshly, even under the cloak of comedy. It's interesting to consider whether today's political climate could support similar satiric approaches. What is perhaps overlooked now is the concept that families can disagree and still show love and commitment to each other.

As spouses face new political battle lines, so do parents and children. A recent study found over 20% of Americans are now estranged from a relative over offensive personal beliefs, which frequently stem from partisan divides (Cox, 2022). Political identity has become intrinsically linked to assessments of personality and moral character. Beliefs on the "other side" signal stupidity, dangerous ignorance, or malicious motivations. Family members rarely grant legitimacy to opposing perspectives, heightening feelings of alienation and rejection.

The ability of parents to pass partisan views to children was previously thought to be relatively high. Recent research, however, indicates that about half of adult children now adopt political affiliations that diverge from their parents' (Hatemi & Ojeda, 2021). Parents offended by children's liberalism or conservatism frequently express feelings of betrayal, confusion, fear, and failure. For some, children not voting "correctly" calls their parenting abilities into question. Children, of course, still seek validation and acceptance of their identities beyond inherited partisan labels. Reminding all family members of reciprocal appreciation for shared connections and unique self-definitions can open pathways for renewed understanding, even with political dissimilarity.

Political differences often exacerbate existing philosophical or cultural gaps particularly between fathers and sons, leading to conflicts over issues like climate change and gender identification. These differences serve to widen the divide on various topics, making it difficult for fathers and sons to connect and understand each other's perspectives. Political disputes can readily become proxies for longstanding personality differences and disappointments (Safer, 2019).

Daughters may influence their fathers' political views, notably around issues of fairness. However, political disputes can provoke anxiety and misunderstandings in father-daughter relationships. Women are increasingly identifying as liberals, which can create stress with conservative fathers, particularly around social issues and deeply held values. While daughters may impact their fathers' perspectives, the dynamics are often different for daughters and mothers. The "relentless hope" trait describes mothers and daughters who cannot accept loved ones' alternate political positions, instead waging indirect campaigns to forcibly transform other's opinions (Safer, 2019). Political disagreements between mothers and daughters often involve more passive-aggressive behaviors and a strong desire to change the other's beliefs. Safer describes this "relentless hope," as the inability to accept differing views within loved ones. These dynamics can lead to heightened tensions and a breakdown in communication. Letting go of the need to politically convert family members allows more tolerance of diversity.

I just couldn't believe that my mother would vote for that man! It's like she was blinded by other's opinions and couldn't see for herself who he is. After a major argument about how she was going to vote in the last election, I just couldn't be around her. That's lasted for 2 years now and I can't seem to forgive her.

(A 24-year-old female college student in Texas)

Sibling Rivalries

Sibling relationships often suffer the most from profound political divides within families. Political arguments easily inflame underlying rivalry and historic parental affection or approval struggles. In some cases, toxic alliances form, with parents and particular offspring uniting against marginalized siblings who embody family scapegoats or outcasts. Siblings might compete for the mantle of most innovative, most successful, or favored child, with political contests becoming the battlefield for lifelong rivalries. Entire branches sever relations over hurtful partisan attacks and power plays. As Safer (2019) notes, political fights are second only to conflicts over aging parents and inheritance in destroying sibling closeness.

What frequently gets lost in political battles between brothers and sisters are the common bonds and history connecting them. Siblings often turn to each other for solace, adventure, and mutual understanding through the formative early years. Now these same siblings only see warped partisan enemies, losing sight of the companions who colored their childhood with laughter and dreams and who warded off "things that go bump in the night." Therapeutic breakthroughs come from identifying this blindness and helping estranged siblings grieve the cherished refuge they once provided each other as innocent playmates. Reconnecting with those joyful memories and enduring qualities of identity beyond politics can start to rebuild broken bridges even between the most polarized siblings.

When there has been a history of conflict or abuse between siblings, the partisan divide can become the battlefield for adult brothers and sisters. Rather than addressing problematic histories, the fight goes on over political issues. The battle for acknowledgement, acceptance, affirmation, and reconciliation sometimes finds a venue in contentious political identities.

In therapy, learning about the history of sibling relationships can guide the focus to those long-standing, unresolved patterns that will need to be addressed if siblings want to work toward reconciliation or letting go.

My older sister was always "the smart one" and was my mother's 'darling girl'. They agreed about a lot of things that I had different beliefs about, like the value of going to college. When I decided after High School to apprentice as a plumber, they were both really upset that I wouldn't be 'educated' enough to have a good life. I became a member of the Republican party when I was eligible to vote, and they were relentless in trying to change my mind. I finally had to tell both of them that if they couldn't shut up about my choices, then they could kiss my ass goodbye. While they've stopped trying to confront me, there's still those 'looks' I get whenever any political topics come up. I just leave the room. I can't wait to move out on my own.

(A 19-year-old male in Florida)

All in the 'Extended' Family

The volatility of extended family political arguments stems from the same good vs. evil moral framing and harsh condemnations seen in other domains of political sectarianism. When cousins, grandparents, aunts, uncles, and in-laws get painted as ignorant racists or godless socialists based solely on voting patterns or yard signs, relationships inevitably rupture. Social media echo chambers further breed self-righteousness and validate extreme caricatures of the political outgroup. Family discussions under these conditions rarely enable nuanced policy debates. Instead, even minor conversations about current events escalate into personal attacks and mutual recriminations.

Because of these types of disputes and tensions, many families dread holiday gatherings due to potential political conflicts. One study documented over 30 million lost hours of Thanksgiving cross-partisan conversation time following the hyper-contentious 2016 U.S. presidential election alone (Chen & Rohla, 2018). Healing politically divided extended families requires abandoning abusive rhetorical patterns of moral condemnation. It also involves embracing bonds of affection and identification that persist beneath partisan identities associated with specific electoral choices or ideologies.

One of the authors met with several clients who experienced this rise in family tensions regarding political differences.

In the early fall of 2023, prior to the holiday season, fully half of the clients I was working with expressed concerns about upcoming family gatherings. This was a topic that previously would arise primarily when there were issues such as family members who drank too much or legacies of highly conflicted divorces. Now, however, the focus of the concern was almost exclusively on political disagreements. Several clients chose to limit their gatherings to immediate family only, others decided to cancel Thanksgiving gatherings altogether. One client, a liberal woman in her 50s, decided that she and her husband would take a short trip away and find a restaurant near their hotel for Thanksgiving dinner to avoid a confrontation with her brother who had become devoted to the Trump "Make America Great Again (MAGA)" movement. This older brother had been her "hero" when she was a child, someone who protected her from an angry father. It was heartbreaking for her to end the tradition of bringing him and his family to join them for Thanksgiving. She stated that "I just can't endure the anger I know will erupt around the table if he's there." Thanksgiving turned into "Thanks, I'm out of here."

Beyond Connection: Families as Complex Systems

Couples or families are not merely collections of individuals. They are intricate systems with unique communication patterns, roles, rules (explicit and unspoken), and emotional processes. These patterns create an internal structure that guides interactions and influences individual behavior. Like many systems, couples and families strive for stability and balance or homeostasis. Even in the early days of dating, couples establish patterns that provide a sense of predictability and security. However, when the system encounters stress, such as a crisis or a significant change, it might fall into chaos. Family theory seeks to understand how families attempt to maintain equilibrium, sometimes even resorting to maladaptive behaviors to do so.

Over time, families develop implicit and often unspoken "scripts" or narratives. These scripts dictate how members should feel, think, and behave. They might be adaptive, leading to healthy interactions, but they can also be limiting and destructive, perpetuating negative or even abusive cycles within the family system.

Many of the most influential dynamics in couples and families operate below the surface of conscious awareness. These may involve the unconscious transmission of patterns, such as unspoken expectations, emotional reactivity, and unresolved issues passed down through generations. They may also involve family of origin influences. Our family of origin (the family we were born into) fundamentally shapes who we become. Patterns we learned as children can unconsciously play out in our adult relationships with our own partners and children. Interpersonal family systems are complex, dynamic entities influenced by a multitude of factors, including sociocultural, economic, and political contexts. Within these systems, political partisanship can often serve as both a surface-level conflict and a means of concealing deeper, more fundamental issues.

Political partisanship within families can serve as a proxy for underlying issues such as unresolved personal conflicts, unmet emotional needs, and long-standing patterns of dysfunctional communication. Families might project these deeper issues onto political disagreements because it provides a tangible, external focus for their tensions. This projection can offer a temporary sense of solidarity within factions of the family, allowing members to form alliances based on shared political beliefs rather than confronting more painful, personal disputes.

Several mechanisms explain how political partisanship conceals deeper family issues. Political arguments allow family members to displace their frustrations and anger from more personal and painful issues to a seemingly less personal, external conflict. Engaging in political debates can be a strategy to avoid addressing more challenging interpersonal issues such as marital discord, parental neglect, substance abuse, affairs, or sibling rivalry. Political partisanship can create scapegoats within the family, where one member is blamed for holding a challenging political view, thus diverting attention from the broader systemic problems within the family. Regular political arguments can become a family ritual, offering a predictable and familiar structure that masks the unpredictability and discomfort of confronting long-standing patterns and emotional issues.

From a structural family therapy perspective, political partisanship can be seen as part of the family's structure, reflecting roles, boundaries, and alliances that are shaped by deeper issues. Political partisanship may define subsystems within the family (e.g., parents vs. children, siblings vs. siblings) and establish boundaries that prevent healthy interaction and problem-solving. From a strategic or more dynamical systems model, political sentiment is often a method that the system uses to regulate the behavior of its members. Political alliances can become coalitions that reinforce power balances and dissipate conflicts, masking underlying issues such as lack of emotional support or unresolved trauma.

There are a variety of overlapping family therapy theories and techniques that are helpful for assisting the highly conflicted partisan family. These include narrative, feminist, psychodynamic, problem-focused, cognitive behavioral, multisystem, intergenerational, and many more. In our experience, strategic family therapy can be especially valuable. It typically focuses on the strategies families use to solve problems, often highlighting how these strategies can become problematic themselves. In the context of political partisanship, families may use ideological differences as a problem-solving strategy to manage stress and conflict, albeit ineffectively. This can involve manipulating alliances and communication patterns to maintain a semblance of harmony. Political conflicts can create feedback loops where the resolution of one argument leads to the emergence of another, perpetuating a cycle of conflict that obscures deeper issues.

Therapists can help families reframe their political conflicts to uncover the underlying issues. For instance, a debate about political ideologies might be reframed as a discussion about unmet needs for respect and validation within the family. Listening for "always" and "never" statements can be a portal to exploring how the current political debate connects to long-standing patterns in a family. When political partisanship abates, it can unmask the issues that were previously concealed. Families may experience an initial sense of relief, but this can quickly give way to the emergence of unresolved conflicts and emotions that had been suppressed. Without the external focus of political partisanship, family members may struggle to navigate these newly exposed issues.

The abatement of political partisanship can remove a common enemy, leading to increased introspection and potential conflict as family members confront their personal and interpersonal issues. The connection of political debates to entrenched patterns of communication can result in emotional flooding, where suppressed feelings and conflicts overwhelm family members, potentially leading to heightened stress and anxiety. Family members who defined their roles and identities through political partisanship may experience confusion and a sense of loss, as they must renegotiate their positions and relationships within the family.

Addressing the history of issues unmasked by the abatement of political partisanship requires a thoughtful and strategic approach. Effective therapeutic interventions are crucial to help families navigate this transition. Therapists can assist by facilitating open communication, promoting empathy, and helping families develop healthier coping strategies. Improving communication skills can be a vital step in addressing the deeper issues concealed by political partisanship. Families often benefit from developing active listening skills to foster empathy and understanding. Techniques as simple as encouraging the use of "I-messages" to express feelings and needs without blame can be genuinely helpful. In more severe cases it is necessary to restructure family roles and boundaries and assist family members in clarifying and negotiating their roles to reduce confusion and power struggles.

Boundaries, Differentiation, and the Politicized Family

Families that are dysfunctional may need intervention that would seem dramatic, perhaps draconian to more non-directive, egalitarian therapists. This often includes setting boundaries. In our experience, some progressive or liberal therapists can be uncomfortable with the seemingly authoritarian stance that setting boundaries in family therapy may require.

Family therapists have long argued that boundary setting is often an important—sometimes quick, sometimes longer term—treatment intervention for a variety of family issues. Therapists who work with politically charged clients can encourage clients to set boundaries on their political activities which can have dramatic effects on partisan beliefs. Limited time spent viewing or listening to 24-hour, partisan "news" sources can be an important step in turning down the level of influence and pervasiveness of exposure to contentious material. Perhaps more compelling is encouraging those in their social networks to limit divisive rhetoric. No more "All liberals/conservatives are idiots" conversations. Practicing civil political conversations with friends and others can help build the skill needed to change patterns with family members.

No one should ever endure verbal abuse from their family, whether rooted in political disagreements or any other topic. Families can best serve as pillars of support and understanding, not sources of hurt and alienation. It is critical that family members communicate differences in opinion with respect and empathy, ensuring that every person feels valued and heard. Promoting an environment where respectful dialogue is the norm and recognizing the inherent worth of each family member, irrespective of their views, are fundamental steps toward building a more compassionate and supportive family dynamic. The case of Susan illustrates this.

Susan

Susan was in therapy because she was involved in a relationship with Mark, a man who gave her minimum attention. She admired his progressive values and his feminist feelings: "What I always wanted in a man." However, he was never available. He was always working on a project for his boss or for people in his community. When he was available, he was often preoccupied with his own events, thoughts, and interests. Although she felt that their relationship "could" work, it wasn't and the numerous requests she had made to Mark were not helpful. Mark just was not who she wanted him to be.

Boundaries for her involved learning to separate respect for her partner's feelings, but not to tolerate his inattention. Eventually, she broke off the relationship and continued to look for someone else. Interestingly, her next partner was more politically conservative, but that did not seem to be a factor in their success as a couple.

For some clients, boundary settings may involve a differentiation of self rather than a return to a historically toxic system. The primary goal of the therapist is to work collaboratively with the family to foster unity and understanding. There are instances, however, when it becomes necessary to encourage family members to differentiate themselves and develop their own interests. This process aligns with principles found in both structural and strategic therapy interventions, emphasizing the importance of balancing family roles and patterns of interaction. In politically charged families, where ideological differences can create significant tension and conflict, promoting differentiation can help individuals maintain their sense of self while navigating complex family dynamics. This strategy is not about fostering estrangement but about enabling individuals to establish healthy boundaries, thereby reducing emotional reactivity and fostering more constructive interactions.

Highly politicized environments often lead to intense emotional fusion, where family members' identities and beliefs become enmeshed. This fusion can result in heightened conflicts, as differing political views are seen not just as opinions but as threats to one's core identity and to family unity. Since partisan behaviors often serve as a distraction from other, unacknowledged issues within the family system, structural therapy interventions focus on reorganizing the family structure to address these dysfunctional patterns. The focus is on helping family members recognize and respect their individual perspectives without feeling threatened by others' differing views. This approach allows family members to engage in discussions about politics and other contentious topics without escalating into destructive arguments. While the therapist works to maintain family cohesion, encouraging differentiation can be a step to preserving the overall family harmony and enabling healthier interactions. Once the partisan behavior is addressed, it is not uncommon for other family problems to surface, revealing deeper relational dynamics that need attention.

In highly politicized families, it is not uncommon for one member to be designated as the identified patient, the person seen as the source of the family's problems. Often, this individual is the one who struggles most with the family's political climate, who outwardly expresses distress, or who engages in political issues that run counter to the family's ideology. By encouraging differentiation, therapists can help shift the focus from scapegoating this identified patient to addressing the broader systemic issues within the family. This approach, central to structural therapy, allows for a more balanced view of the family's dynamics and fosters collective responsibility for maintaining healthy relationships. It helps each member see how their behaviors contribute to the overall family system, thus reducing undue blame on the identified patient and promoting a more supportive family environment.

Differentiation helps family members develop greater emotional resilience, which is essential for maintaining a balanced family dynamic. In politicized families, individuals often feel pressured to conform to the dominant family viewpoint, leading to suppressed emotions and unresolved tensions. Strategic therapy interventions can be employed to disrupt these rigid patterns and introduce more flexible, adaptive behaviors. Encouraging family members to differentiate helps them articulate their thoughts and feelings openly, without fear of rejection or conflict. This process not only fosters personal growth but also enhances the family's ability to manage conflicts constructively. Each member learns to appreciate diverse perspectives within the family, leading to a more supportive and understanding environment. The therapist's role is to guide this process, helping the family see the value in each member's unique viewpoint. By addressing the underlying issues that emerge once partisan behaviors are managed, therapists can help families achieve a more profound and lasting resolution.

Differentiation is particularly important in preventing the entrenchment of polarized thinking within families, which can undermine family cohesion. When family members are too closely enmeshed, political differences can become a source of persistent stress and anxiety. By encouraging differentiation, therapists help individuals detach from the immediate emotional reactions that such differences might provoke. This detachment does not mean disinterest or lack of concern, but rather the ability to engage with differing viewpoints thoughtfully, respectfully, and without undue emotional turmoil. This skill is central to fostering a more nuanced and empathetic understanding of each other's perspectives, thereby strengthening the family's cohesive bonds while also recognizing the importance of individual growth. This process also prepares the family to handle the new issues that may arise once the focus on partisan conflict is reduced.

Furthermore, differentiation allows family members to develop and assert their own values and beliefs independently, which is essential for maintaining healthy family dynamics. In politically charged families, the pressure to align with the predominant family ideology can stifle individual development and self-expression. By encouraging differentiation, therapists support individuals in exploring and affirming their own political beliefs, leading to a more authentic and satisfying sense of self. This self-assuredness can reduce the likelihood of internal conflict and improve overall mental well-being. The therapist helps family members see that by pursuing their own interests and beliefs, they can still contribute positively to the family. As family members become more differentiated, underlying issues previously masked by political conflict may come to light, offering new opportunities for growth and healing.

Another significant benefit of promoting differentiation in politicized families is the enhancement of communication skills, which are crucial for maintaining family cohesion. When family members can maintain their individuality, they are better equipped to engage in open and honest dialogue. Differentiation fosters an environment where members feel safe to express their thoughts and feelings without fear of retribution or rejection. This openness is crucial for resolving conflicts and building mutual understanding, as it encourages listening and empathy. Improved communication can help bridge the gaps created by political differences, allowing families to find common ground and shared values despite their ideological diversity. The therapist's role is to facilitate these conversations, ensuring they are constructive and respectful. With the removal of partisan behaviors, new communication patterns can emerge, and addressing previously unspoken family issues is possible.

Therapists also recognize that promoting differentiation can help in addressing deeper, underlying issues that may be masked by political conflicts, which can be crucial for family cohesion. Often, intense political disagreements within families are symptomatic of broader relational problems, such as unresolved past conflicts, power struggles, or unmet emotional needs. By encouraging family members to differentiate, therapists help them uncover and address these root issues. This process leads to more profound healing and a stronger, more resilient family structure. Members learn to support each other's growth and well-being, which can diminish the impact of political disagreements. When partisan behaviors are reduced, the family often confronts these deeper issues, providing an opportunity for significant progress.

Finally, differentiation can prevent the long-term negative impacts of political partisanship on family relationships. Without proper boundaries, political disagreements can erode the foundational bonds of love and respect within a family. Therapists, by promoting differentiation, help family members build a healthier relational dynamic where differences are accepted and valued rather than being a source of division. This approach ultimately strengthens the family unit, ensuring that political diversity does not overshadow the fundamental connections that bind family members together. By focusing on individual growth and mutual respect, therapists help politicized families navigate their differences while maintaining strong, loving relationships. In this way, differentiation supports lasting family cohesion, despite the challenges of a highly politicized environment, by empowering each member to develop their own interests and identities. This, in turn, allows the family to address and resolve other issues that may have been previously overshadowed by political conflict.

Helping Families Build Better Connections

Healing politically divided family relationships requires abandoning abusive rhetorical patterns of moral condemnation. It also involves embracing bonds of affection and identification that persist beneath partisan identities associated with specific political choices or ideologies. Facilitating open, nonjudgmental dialogues focused on understanding divergent experiences and values differentiating family members can foster reconciliation. Individuals ultimately must let go of wanting to politically convert kin, instead accepting legitimate diversity and pluralism as a foundation for renewed family connection. At times the family therapist may need to be firm in insisting on these rules.

Mental health professionals and clients can benefit from guidelines for discussing politics within families. These include setting intentions, practicing active and reflective listening, showing respect, focusing on other aspects of the relationship, staying calm, and knowing when to stop. These strategies can help families navigate political discussions without damaging their relationships. Facilitating open, nonjudgmental dialogues which focus on understanding the divergent experiences and values of different family members can foster respect and possibly reconciliation. Individuals ultimately must let go of wanting to politically convert kin, instead accepting legitimate diversity and pluralism as a foundation for renewed family connection.

Counselors and therapists can lower the volume of partisan bickering by unplugging from highly polarized media and encouraging clients to do the same. We can also seek out diverse perspectives on social and political issues and encourage our clients to do the same.

We offer some suggestions based on clinical experience:

- Help clients contextualize political debates by therapeutically exploring influences behind beliefs like family background, emotional experiences, and cohort events.

- When assessments turn personal, shift the focus back to multidimensional identities and shared positive qualities that attract and bond partners and family members.
- Teach crucial interpersonal skills like reflective listening, emotionally focused dialogues, self-soothing techniques, and tolerance of disagreement and uncertainty. Often, counselors and therapists minimize these skills because they are part of our framework. However, to clients who have not mastered them, they can be remarkable.
- Explore family triangulation and role dynamics that might be exacerbating polarization as displacement for deeper emotional conflicts between members.
- Convey nonjudgmental understanding for all positions—political beliefs often serve unmet psychological needs for safety, belonging, autonomy, and competence.
- Refer clients to educational resources (like Braver Angels depolarization skills workshops and the Couple CARE program; see Appendix A) for practical training in overcoming political divides that are threatening key relationships.

Summary

This chapter reviewed research detailing how political sectarianism currently impacts romantic, parent-child, and extended family relationships. Politicized reasons for increased dating selectivity, couple dissatisfaction, and family estrangements were examined, highlighting the role of moral stereotypes and judgments attached to partisan labels in driving interpersonal tensions. Building motivation for mutual understanding and acceptance across political differences, while also nurturing positive shared connections, provides a pathway to mitigate relational harms resulting from destructive polarization. Mental health professionals play crucial roles supporting this societal reconciliation one relationship at a time through therapeutic alliances.

References

Change Research. (2023, September 18) *Young women are more liberal than young men.* https://changeresearch.com/post/young-women-are-more-liberal-than-young-men/

Chen, M. C. & Rohla, R. (2018, June 1). The effect of partisanship and political advertising on close family ties. *Science, 360*(6392), 1020–1024. https://doi.org/10.1126/science.aaq1433

Cox, D. A. (2022, February 9). *Emerging trends and enduring patterns in American family life.* American Enterprise Institute: The Survey Center on American Life. www.americansurveycenter.org/research/emerging-trends-and-enduring-patterns-in-american-family-life; www.conservativetherapists.com/

Gottman, J. M., & Silver, N. (2015). *The seven principles for making marriage work: A practical guide from the country's foremost relationship expert*. New York, NY: Three Rivers Press.

Guralnik, O. (2023, May 16). *I'm a couple therapist. Something new is happening in relationships*. The New York Times Magazine: The Therapy Issue.

Hatemi, P. K. & Ojeda, C. (2021, July). The role of child perception and motivation in political socialization. *British Journal of Political Science, 51*(3).

Match.com MediaRoom. (2020, October 6). *Match releases 10th annual singles in America survey, revealing how 2020 has transformed dating*. https://match.mediaroom.com/2020-10-06-Match-Releases-10th-Annual-Singles-in-America-Survey-Revealing-How-2020-Has-Transformed-Dating?printable

Peacock, C. & Pederson, J. R. (2022, May 10). Love and politics: The influence of politically (dis)similar romantic relationships on political participation and relationship satisfaction. *Human Communication Research, 48*(4), 567–578. https://doi.org/10.1093/hcr/hqac011

Safer, J. (2019). *I love you, but I hate your politics: How to protect your intimate relationships in a poisonous partisan world*. London: Biteback Publishing.

Sauerheber, J. D., Hughey, A. W., Wolf, C. P., Ginn, B., & Stethen, A. (2021). The relationship among and between marital satisfaction, religious faith, and political orientation. *The Family Journal, 29*(1), 41–49. https://doi.org/10.1177/1066480720939023

Survey Center on American Life. (2022, May 31). *The growing political divide between young men and women*. Survey Center on American Life. https://americansurveycenter.org

11

DEPOLARIZATION, TRAINING, AND SUPPORT

Depolarization: The Foundation of Effective Work Across the Political Divide

For clinicians, depolarization training is important to assure that we can work effectively with clients across the political spectrum. Depolarizing means we distinguish between positions and people, and we appreciate that political views are complicated. We accept our own reactivity when we hear something that is challenging to us and stay aware of what signals we may be sending to the client. If we hold the view that people on the other side are idiots, ignorant, or evil, then we begin to listen and react to them in a different way. In her Ted Talk "On Being Wrong" (March, 2011), Kathryn Schulz describes how attached we are to the idea that our thoughts and beliefs are an ideal reflection of reality. She suggests that the "miracle of our mind is that we can see the world as it isn't" (Schulz, 2011). It reminds us to be humble and practice humility when we encounter world views different from those we hold dear. In her book, "I Never Thought of It That Way" (2022b), Monica Guzman asks: "What is keeping us from seeing each other, and how do we get it (the hell) out of our way?" (p. xxv). Polarization appears to be the problem and part of the solution is depolarization.

What do we mean by "depolarization"? It's a term that may be unfamiliar to many clinicians, but it is a crucial concept to understand when working with highly politicized people. Polarization is a process that is characterized by an individuals' political views moving toward more extreme positions. The further from the middle we move, the more polarized we become. All of us fall somewhere along a continuum of what we feel positive toward and what we have a negative view of when considering a wide variety of social and political issues. Most people are

DOI: 10.4324/9781032651217-11

somewhere near the middle and "lean" to one side or the other regarding how we should best address a wide array of political and social problems. Polarization begins when we lose respect or appreciation for different perspectives. We begin to believe that those who disagree with us do not hold reasonable, intelligent, thoughtful ideas. There is a barrier to appreciating the contributions that those who disagree with us can offer in creating solutions to shared problems.

Polarization is not simply a differing set of beliefs, it encompasses a variety of thoughts and actions that divide people into categories of "with me" or "against me." It's a process of categorizing people or opinions into completely opposing groups. The more polarized a person becomes, the more they view those who have other perspectives as enemies. Most of us have seen our political discourse getting much worse; more combative and dismissive of those with whom we don't agree. Over the past several decades our government, at both a local and national level, has become polarized to the point of being unable to function effectively. When we consider someone an enemy, the dynamic is focused on winning or on eliminating them rather than finding common ground and working together toward solutions.

From neighborhood school board meetings to the halls of Congress, our inability to come together across party lines has become a threat to our very existence as a functioning democracy. When we're confronted with problems that need resolution, democracies rely on having multiple viewpoints represented. Neither side has all the answers or a "perfect" solution. Negotiating in good faith among diverse people with different perspectives is the foundation of a representative government at all levels; democracy cannot exist for long without cooperation.

> In over two centuries, there has been no democracy without political parties. When public confidence in political parties is compromised, the entire democratic process suffers. In all sustainable democracies, the party system must be deeply and durably entrenched in the fabric of society.
>
> *(National Democratic Institute, 2008)*

A functioning democracy is built on and maintained by the ideas, backgrounds, and experiences of a broad coalition of people.

In 2008, the National Democratic Institute (NDI) published a document titled, "Minimum Standards for the Democratic Functioning of Political Parties." The following section highlights the importance of respect and cooperation between opposing viewpoints:

Respect for Other Parties and Free Competition

All democratic parties have a right to expect that they and their supporters may freely express their opinions; governing parties and state institutions have an obligation to protect these rights, and to safeguard the environment of free competition. Political parties should demonstrate their commitment to democratic decision making by showing respect for other parties and other interests in society. Parties, particularly those in government, should recognize that other parties and groups, as well as individual citizens, all have the right to peacefully challenge and oppose them. This means that however fiercely parties campaign, they will not question the rights of others to defend their interests and promote their principles, provided those opponents work within the recognized democratic framework. It means that legislative parties will deal with all other elected representatives and will recognize their mandates and their rights to take legislative seats. It means that governing parties will not use government resources or legislative authority in ways that make it impossible for other voices to be heard (for instance, by imposing media censorship). Parties may fervently disagree with each other, but at the very least they must tolerate their democratic opponents; of course, parties may even welcome most such disputes as being a key component of democratic politics.

(NDI, 2008, p. 3)

We see the impact of large numbers of people in the United States, and in many other countries around the world, who have become deeply polarized politically and socially. The threat and use of violence, angry and dismissive rhetoric aimed at each other, and the belief that the other side is threatening to destroy our country has taken hold of many of our citizens on both sides of the aisle. Regardless of whether we are liberal or conservative, there is a much stronger vein of polarization in our relationship to those on the other side. Doherty (2022) describes the "rise over several decades of social (or affective) polarization where ordinary Americans have come to regard people who vote differently as untrustworthy enemies" (p. 137). We are far beyond seeing the other side as an "opponent"; someone who has different views and ideas but is worthy of appreciation and engagement. When people are seen as the enemy, they become unworthy of attempts at connection. They are "idiots" who refuse to see "reality." At best they need to be avoided or silenced, and at worst, eliminated. At every level, from our intimate partners, to our neighborhood, to our country, we see the impact of the trend toward exclusion and disconnection.

At the Illinois Republican State Convention on June 16, 1858, Abraham Lincoln built his speech around the Bible verse (Mark 3:35) that states "And if a house be divided against itself, that house cannot stand" (Fehrenbacher, 1960). At that time in our history, the issue that divided the country was slavery and the Civil War was largely fought to determine whether the United States would truly be a free country for all men and women who resided in its borders. Currently, the rhetoric that divides us has become more focused on seeing the other side as immoral, anti-American, dangerous, and untrustworthy. The divide has moved beyond debate about the issues that divide us, like immigration and abortion, and has become more directed at the character and intentions of those on the other side of the aisle. We are losing a sense of connection to a common purpose and to respectful discourse regarding our differences and how to address our concerns. The United States of America resembles the "Divided States" of Lincoln's era.

> Since the rise of "Trumpism", I've seen this shift in so many of my liberal friends, colleagues, and clients. Typically, conservatives are described as "ignorant", "misguided", "idiots", and sometimes "evil". There is often a refusal to engage in even routine social exchanges with someone who identifies as a Republican. I've had both patients and friends decline social invitations from conservative neighbors or family members and even sell their homes and move to an area where they're less likely to encounter people with different political perspectives. There's an increased avoidance and rejection of opportunities to interact or build relationships with politically diverse people that is far more common than I've encountered in the past. We seem to be seeking refuge from those with whom we don't agree. We're becoming an increasingly divided country. It feels to me as though our house is shaking on its foundations.
>
> *(A 72-year-old psychologist in Florida)*

As we've explored in other chapters, there are both "nurture" and "nature" aspects at work beginning early in our lives that build a foundation of moral values which guide the development of our world view and political leanings. These views are not predetermined, but we are predisposed to embrace certain beliefs and approaches to experience that are reflected in our political affiliations. That doesn't mean, however, that we can't engage in discourse, appreciate the contributions of those on the other side of the spectrum, and work cooperatively to address the issues and concerns that we share. We always will have differences politically, but we don't have to become polarized. Ezra Klein's (2020) book "Why We're Polarized" is a fascinating history of how we've reached our current level of division and distrust over the past 50 years in the United States. He summarizes that in the last five decades, on both sides, we've become more likely to vote for "our party" than the candidate, not because we like our party so much, but because we dislike the opposing party more. "Even as hope and change sputter, fear and loathing proceed" (Klein, 2020, p. 10).

It's inevitable that this partisanship and polarization will increasingly be a factor in the therapy space. In conversations with our colleagues, both authors have encountered professionals who are unwilling to work with clients who have a political orientation different than their own. In informal interviews, we've heard polarizing rhetoric from both sides. Here are a few samples we've collected.

- *"She came in because she was depressed. But her real problem was she was a whiney wannabe snowflake liberal."*
- *"As soon as I learned he (the potential client) had voted for Trump, I told him he'd need to find another therapist."*
- *"I just don't feel comfortable working with someone who has such poor moral values and stupid political views."*

As noted, we believe that it's critical to include information on political depolarization in our cross-cultural and diversity training and with continuing education offerings. We need to be able to recognize and effectively manage our own biases and reactivity and build therapeutic relationships that avoid stereotypes, ridicule, and dismissiveness. Let's explore how we challenge our biases and learn to depolarize.

How Do We Depolarize?

There are steps that we can take to depolarize ourselves so that we can more effectively work with clients who are on the other side of the political divide. While specific training may focus more on different aspects of depolarizing, we believe that the following components are an integral part of learning this skill. These are the criteria that are important for mental health professionals to look for in depolarization training:

- Understanding and acknowledging our biases
- Developing "radical curiosity"
- Practicing communication skills
- Demonstrating respect and appreciation
- Accessing resources for information, training, and support

Understanding and Acknowledging Our Biases

We begin the process of depolarization by acknowledging that we carry biases and beliefs that impact our work with others. Like religious and cultural beliefs, our political orientations are often a core part of what defines who we are and the values that guide us. Thinking that we are a "blank slate" is a concept that can make us more vulnerable to ineffective, even harmful interactions with our clients. Most clinicians are aware of how our body language, tone of voice, avoidance of certain topics, and other behaviors can impact our work. We spend a great deal of time training therapists to become familiar with the unintended signals we send when we're uncomfortable or triggered by a client. We have many reactions, often non-verbal, that indicate we're annoyed, distressed, or upset. Our facial expressions, tone of voice, eye contact and other "tells" are difficult to control when we hear something that we find offensive. Clients are often especially tuned in to how we're responding, and those subtle physical communications often significantly impact our work together. If you are skeptical about this phenomenon, watch what happens when you can't stifle a yawn during a session.

Cheryl Dolinger Brown, LCSW, provides a workshop for mental health professionals titled: "Bridging the Divide: Developing Relationships Between People with Diverse Views" (Brown, 2023). She usually starts her workshop by inquiring, "Who don't you want to listen to?" It's an elegant way to bring our attention to those clients who present a challenge to our values. To effectively depolarize, we must acknowledge that we have biases and be willing to work to minimize their impact on our clients. It doesn't mean we erase our beliefs, but we work to become more aware of how we react when we're triggered and, hopefully, we build a tolerance for being uncertain. We stay open to information that doesn't correspond with what we believe is true or right.

We can tell we're triggered by politically based statements from others when we become judgmental and see the other person as ignorant or misguided. Bias tends to build a frame around how we view the person based on their beliefs or opinions. When we have a negative reaction to someone's political positions, that negative frame can become filled with our biases and influence our perspective on many aspects of that person's life. If they believe that, can they be a good parent? Are they able to make reasonable, rational choices? Polarization means we're stuck in feeling that our beliefs are always correct and are an objective reflection of reality. We become attached to our own "righteousness." People who are politically polarized are not using their reasoning mind to search for truth, they are "reasoning in support of their emotional reactions" (Haidt, 2012, p. 29). Acknowledging our biases is the foundation for managing them effectively in the counseling relationship.

Developing "Radical Curiosity"

Where do we start opening our eyes and ears to the world that we don't know? Monica Guzman, a journalist, author, and Senior Fellow for Public Practice with Braver Angels (https://braverangels.org/) advocates for "radical curiosity" in her Ted Talk, "How Curiosity Will Save Us" (Guzman, 2022a). She describes curiosity as the gap between what you know and what you want to know. The question Guzman encourages us to ask ourselves is "What am I missing?" (Guzman, 2022a, p. 48). We learn to question our certainty that we have the "correct" way of understanding the world. We understand that we see reality not as it is, but as we are. Guzman believes that when we avoid people with whom we disagree, we miss a chance to learn something and get a more complex understanding of a problem. She asks; "What kinds of people do I talk about, but not with?" (Guzman, 2022a).

Turning assumptions into questions is how we initiate radical curiosity when engaged with someone who sees the world differently. The questions to explore with them are:

1. How (not why) did you come to believe what you believe?
2. What are your hopes and concerns?
3. What do you care about most?

Guzman (2022b) encourages us to use curiosity to pursue "INTOIT's": "I Never Thought Of It That way" moments. It's an experience that therapists are particularly familiar with; that encounter with a client that changes your understanding of something. We can only learn something new from others who have different life experiences than we do. Our curiosity is the link to connection with others; it opens the door to a different perspective. Guzman's "curiosity starter kit" has four steps: 1. Mind the gap, 2. Collect knowledge, 3. Reject easy answers, and 4. Embrace complexity (Guzman, 2022b, p. 62). It's a good formula for approaching people with different world views. First, "mind the gap" by appreciating what you don't know: that's the origin of curiosity. Second, "collect knowledge" by asking about other's beliefs and perspectives. Do some research into world views different than yours and expose yourself to some new perspective. Third, "reject easy answers" by focusing not on others, but on your own beliefs and the certainty that you are "right." Challenge your perspectives and move beyond simplification of other's perspectives. Fourth and finally, embrace complexity and all the confusion and uncertainty that come with the chaos of challenging what we know. We're all familiar with the experience of doing complicated things that become more interesting as we learn more. "In a lot of ways, confusion is just complexity before you put curiosity to work" (Guzman, 2022b, p. 70).

Practicing Communication Skills

When clients seek help for problems in their relationships, they almost inevitably state that "We just can't communicate." Training therapists in communication skills is essential to our competence as practitioners because they are necessary for us to build a working relationship with clients. Research has consistently supported how critical it is to the therapeutic relationship for us to establish an empathic, supportive connection (Lambert, 1992). We are always encountering others who are different from us in some ways, but when another's ideas challenge our cherished beliefs and opinions, it becomes more difficult to listen without judgment. This is especially true when we feel that our values are being challenged. I trust that all practitioners have had experiences with clients who strike a nerve by sharing something that goes against our deeply held values. We struggle with how to best respond in a way that preserves the therapeutic relationship. How do we stay in that accepting and emotionally intimate space when we're triggered by something a client shares? We learn and practice our communication skills.

The communication skill that is usually at the root of misunderstandings is the ability to listen with an open mind. Active listening is a foundational skill for the work that we do. In the "Depolarizing Within" trainings that are offered through Braver Angels (https://braverangels.org), they teach **LAPP Skills** which are Listen, Acknowledge, Pivot, and Perspective.

Listen: Listen for the other person's values and emotions that trigger us. Pay attention to what experiences the other person has had that may have formed those beliefs and whether there's a deeper story there. Listening with curiosity is what guides us and helps us manage our own reactions. An example of a question is: "I'm curious how you came to believe _____?"

Acknowledge: Express empathy and concern for what's being shared. The skill of reflective listening is the foundation of acknowledging what you've heard. Approaching the client from an "I hear you …" perspective is the basis for empathy. Stick with it until the client feels heard. An example is: "I understand that your concerns about _____ come from your experiences with _____."

Pivot: A pivot is a shift in the conversation in which you share some of your perspective in a way that builds connection with someone who has a different viewpoint. While this is used in social situations, therapists should always assess whether to bring themselves into the conversation with a client. Like any other self-disclosure, it can help to build trust if we're more transparent with the client about our political leanings. Pivoting is best used if the client introduces a politicized topic. Some clients will ask directly about your positions regarding politics and social issues, and some will not be interested. As noted in Chapter 4, adding information about how you approach political discussions in your profile information may encourage clients to share any concerns they have related to these topics.

The most important guideline for a pivot is to use "I statements" and to only share what the client is interested in hearing. An example of a pivot is: "I agree with your concerns about what is going on, it's something that I have also tried to better understand. Our beliefs or experiences may be different, but I think that complicated issues are best understood when we have a variety of perspectives to draw from." The client may want to hear more, but let that request come from them. It's important that this not be an attempt on the clinicians' part to try and persuade the client to accept your viewpoint or debate the topic.

Perspective: If you do share your thoughts or beliefs with a client, commenting on your perspective can be another way to build trust in the relationship. The goal here is to build respect and communication skills with the client that they can then use in other social interactions. Perspective comments can include:

- Not everyone on either side thinks the same way.
- It's complicated and there are many ways to approach a problem.
- We come to our beliefs from different backgrounds and experiences.
- Neither side has all the answers.
- I believe in the importance of mutual respect.

Examples of perspective statements are: "I'm interested in learning more about the your beliefs, especially those that are different than mine", "I've come to believe that we can better determine how to solve problems when we commit to being respectful and learning to listen to each other", "I don't think that either side of this issue has all the answers to this problem", or "I believe that we're more likely to find solutions when we work together".

With some clients, the Pivot and Perspective aspects of this model may not be a part of the therapy. For clients who are highly defensive, especially sensitive to rejection, or uninterested in hearing your perspective, simply stick to Listen and Acknowledge skills. As described in previous chapters, clients are increasingly bringing these topics into the therapy space, and many are aware that most mental health professionals have a liberal orientation. With clients who are curious about your beliefs, the Pivot and Perspective skills may help to respond in a way that builds greater trust and mutual respect.

Demonstrating Respect and Appreciation

The LAPP model that is the core of depolarizing trainings developed by Braver Angels is a model for demonstrating respect and building appreciation for other viewpoints. The divide that we're experiencing now in our politics has always been with us and always will be so long as we have a functioning democracy in the United States. Through respectful dialogue, whether with clients, colleagues, or friends, we can lower the levels of mistrust, fear, and anger that currently characterize so many interactions about politics and social issues. As psychotherapists, we can build stronger therapeutic alliances with those who bring divergent beliefs to therapy sessions.

Demonstrating respect and appreciation starts with our commitment to learn and practice the skills that help us connect with those who see the world very differently than we do. We can appreciate that we don't have all the answers, and that cooperation and negotiation strengthen us and provide better solutions. Everyone wants to be heard, understood, and accepted: people often seek therapy to have those experiences. Depolarization is a pragmatic approach to help us and those we serve to move forward and build better connections. A Braver Angels workshop participant stated: *"Neither side is going to vanquish the other, so we better figure out how to get along and run the country together"* (Braver Angels, Depolarizing Within Participant Guide, p. 6).

When we go through the process of depolarizing, we move through several stages:

- Hate or fear: They are enemies out to destroy our way of life.
- Disdain: They are ignorant idiots and should know better.
- Pity: The are well meaning but duped or misinformed.
- Basic Respect: They make contributions even if they are mostly off base.
- Respect and Appreciation: They make unique and necessary contributions.

(Braver Angels, 2022, p. 1)

Not all of us start with hatred or fear and not all of us reach a level of respect and appreciation. We believe, however, that pursuing a better understanding of the beliefs and positions of those on the other side of the divide can make us more effective overall as therapists. All of us have our limits and we need to take care of ourselves if we're confronted by a client who is hostile or threatening. None of us can work with everyone we encounter. However, the more informed and better trained we are, the wider the circle of people we can serve.

Essentially, we can't work effectively with someone that we think is an "idiot." Our clients, like ourselves, are an imperfect mixture of contradictory beliefs, ideas, opinions, impulses, and desires. Our goal as psychotherapists is not to dissuade others from their beliefs, but to help them become more authentic, integrated, effective, and connected individuals and members of their communities. Respect and appreciation are the foundations that help us to assist and support others in moving their lives in that direction.

Finding Information, Training, and Support

When political or social issues arise in the therapy space, how can we continue to improve our knowledge and skills to establish and maintain an effective therapeutic relationship? Fortunately, there are organizations, workshops, discussion groups, and other resources that are addressing the need to help us depolarize so that we can effectively connect to those across the political divide. For the mental health professions to remain relevant and respected, we must commit to welcoming people from across the spectrum of political beliefs into our therapy space.

As mental health professionals we have a commitment to seek out research, information, and connection with teaching or training resources when developing new skills in working with unfamiliar issues or populations. The resources for information, engagement, training, and support provided in Appendix B are all established, well-respected, and readily available to those who want to learn how to best bridge the political divide. From our own experience, we know it can be challenging to learn to depolarize and open ourselves to encounters with people with whom we disagree. What's clear, however, is that it's benefited us personally and professionally and helped us to be better citizens and therapists. We trust that you'll experience that as well when you engage with and learn from others who are on that path.

Summary

We believe it is important for therapists to develop skills in assisting politically diverse clients so that our professions don't alienate or isolate individuals who hold diverse views about social issues and politics. Depolarization is a skill set that we can learn and incorporate into our work which is helpful both to the client and to us. Depolarization allows us to become less reactive and more accepting and respectful of others who have a very different political and world view than ours. This is helpful in being a more effective therapist and, we believe, in being a better citizen. This chapter also encourages our colleagues to access a variety of resources and support networks and seek consultation and support to assist in our work with politically challenging clients.

References

Braver Angels. (2022). *Depolarizing within participant guide.* https://braverangels.org/
Brown, C. D. (2023). *Bridging the divide: Developing relationships between people with diverse views.* soulwisdom@aol.com .
Doherty, W. J. (2022). *The ethical lives of clients: Transcending self-interest in psychotherapy.* Washington, DC: American Psychological Association.
Fehrenbacher, D. E. (1960). The origins and purpose of Lincoln's 'House-Divided' speech. *Mississippi Valley Historical Review, 46*(4), 615–643. https://doi.org/10.2307/1886280
Guzman, M. (2022a, February 1). *How curiosity will save us.* Ted Talks, Seattle. www.ted.com/talks/jonathan_haidt_how_common_threats_can_make_common_political_ground?utm_campaign=tedspread&utm_medium=referral&utm_source=tedcomshare

Guzman, M. (2022b). *I never thought of it that way: How to have fearlessly curious conversations in dangerously divided times.* Dallas, TX: BenBella Books, Inc.

Haidt, J. (2012). *The righteous mind: Why good people are divided by politics and religion.* New York, NY: Vintage.

Klein, E. (2020). *Why we're polarized.* New York, NY: Avid Reader Press.

Lambert, M. J. (1992). Psychotherapy outcome research: Implications for integrative and eclectic therapists. In J. C. Norcross & M. R. Goldfried (Eds.), *Handbook of psychotherapy.*

National Democratic Institute (NDI). (2008). *Minimum standards for the democratic functioning of political parties.* Washington, DC: National Democratic Institute. www.ndi.org/sites/default/files/2337_partynorms_engpdf_07082008.pdf

Schulz, K. (March, 2011). *On being wrong.* Ted Talk. www.ted.com/talks/kathryn_schulz _on_being_wrong?subtitle=en

12

ETHICS AND ADVOCACY

Beyond Ordinary Ethics

To effectively treat highly partisan clients, mental health therapists must engage ethically and effectively in candid self-reflection about their own political views, biases, and strongly held emotional responses to hot-button issues. A therapist who fails to acknowledge their leanings may be more prone to countertransference that interferes with the treatment. Like our religious/spiritual beliefs, our political leanings are often a central part of how we view the world and those we encounter. When someone shares that "I voted for ____ " that translates into learning something significant about them and their values. The name that fills the blank in that sentence is likely to produce either a sense of familiarity and bonding or a negative reaction ranging from mild distaste to outright rejection. It's not unusual to encounter colleagues who have stated that "I won't work with anyone who voted for____." Is that refusal to work with someone because of their politics ethical?

Examining one's views can also help the therapist cultivate genuine empathy for a client's political fervor, even when they disagree with the client's ideology. Most people who are drawn to partisan extremes are motivated by an idealistic desire to make the world better—a desire the therapist likely shares. However, their vision of positive change may look quite different from the therapist's. Reflecting on this common ground of basic human yearning for justice and progress can foster compassion.

At the same time, self-reflection should heighten the therapist's vigilance for potential collusion with a partisan client's more unhealthy, destructive or inaccurate beliefs. A therapist who has strong political opinions must be

DOI: 10.4324/9781032651217-12

scrupulously mindful not to let confirmation bias creep in when a client expresses views that align with their own. Regularly consulting with colleagues for outside perspectives is valuable as is training designed to manage political polarization in ourselves.

Another practical ethic involves avoiding stereotyping, which is much more difficult than many clinicians imagine. When a client presents with extreme ideological views, it can be tempting for the therapist to make assumptions about what other beliefs, traits or behaviors will accompany that partisan stance. People are complex and often embody seeming contradictions. It's important not to pigeonhole partisan clients or relate to them as one-dimensional caricatures.

Not all clients with far-left views will fit the stereotype of a "bleeding heart liberal," just as not all far-right clients will match the "red-necked conservative" trope. Partisan clients may surprise the therapist with the nuance of their perspectives. Even when they express opinions the therapist disagrees with, these opinions often arise from a place of sincere good intentions. Approaching each client as a unique individual guards against ethical lapses.

The key is to remain ever mindful of one's own biases and reactions, differentiate between ideological views and problematic behaviors, calibrate confrontation carefully, focus on underlying emotions and needs rather than surface content, and uphold firm boundaries to ensure that extremism does not undermine the safety and integrity of the therapy. With this foundation, mental health therapists can help partisan clients lead more fulfilling lives.

Another crucial aspect involves managing the use of the self in therapy. When discussing politically charged issues with partisan clients, mental health therapists must thoughtfully utilize their own perspectives to preserve the integrity of the therapeutic relationship. Especially when there are strong disagreements, it is important for the client to feel the relationship is a safe haven, not a place where they will be judged, debated, or indoctrinated.

This does not mean the therapist has to be a blank slate devoid of opinions or reactions. Judiciously bringing the therapist's perspective into the room can foster a healthy back-and-forth and provide modeling for the client on how to engage with different views respectfully. If a client says something blatantly false, cruel, or dangerous, gently pushing back may be clinically indicated. The therapist should be thoughtful about the purpose and likely impact of such self-disclosures and always keep the client's needs front and center. Challenging a partisan client's view should be done sparingly and only in service of therapeutic goals, not in service of the therapist's ego or need to be "right." Timing, tact, and framing are key.

For example, suppose a client with far-right or perhaps even moderately conservative views, complains that immigrants are "invading" the country and driving up crime rates. This is a common sentiment in many clients with a more right-leaning perspective. In that case, the therapist might neutrally share some objective crime statistics demonstrating that immigration does not increase crime. However, this should be followed by empathetic curiosity about the client's fear, and exploration of how this fear might be harming the client even if it feels protective to them.

The therapist must also set clear boundaries around behaviors that create an unsafe or hostile environment in therapy. If a client is using slurs, denigrating the therapist's own identity, or refusing to engage in treatment, the therapist should assertively explain that such conduct is unacceptable and outline consequences. Partisan views must not be allowed to impede the actual work of therapy.

Ethical Principles: The Big Five

As a mental health therapist, maintaining ethical standards is essential when working with all clients. Additional considerations come into play when clients hold extreme ideological views on the far left or far right of the political spectrum. The key ethical concepts explored in this chapter are the principles of beneficence, non-maleficence, autonomy, justice, and fidelity, which are the core concepts of the code of ethics in our various disciplines (Dyer, Kohrt, & Candilis, 2021).

The ethical principles in mental health disciplines share a common core, rooted in a shared philosophical tradition spanning from ancient times through the Enlightenment and into the 20th century (Mishna, Underwood, Milne, & Gibson, 2013). These principles are often framed by the concepts of **Beneficence** (doing good) and **Non-Maleficence** (avoiding harm), which, while independent, are deeply interconnected. A mental health professional, whether a therapist or any other practitioner, may find themselves in situations where they do both good and harm to a client. Nonetheless, the overarching ethical goal is to maximize good while minimizing harm.

This ethical balancing act becomes especially challenging when working with highly politicized clients. When a client expresses extreme or fringe views, therapists must carefully navigate the dual responsibilities of helping the client and avoiding the reinforcement of harmful beliefs or behaviors. This delicate balance underscores the shared ethical commitment across mental health disciplines to promote well-being and prevent harm, even in the face of complex and politically charged situations.

For example, if a client with far-left views expresses prejudice, antagonism or dehumanizing attitudes toward more conservative groups, the counselor must be careful not to inadvertently reinforce or validate those views in an effort to develop rapport and trust with the client. At the same time, challenging such views too directly could undermine the therapeutic relationship and the therapist's ability to help the client. Throughout this volume, we have argued that counselors and therapists must strike a delicate balance—listening to the client with empathy to understand the underlying emotions, fears, and life experiences that fuel extreme views while still firmly holding the line against hate, prejudice, and the endorsement of violence. Shifting the focus to the client's pain and unmet needs, rather than arguing over ideology itself, is often most productive.

Our view is that in almost all cases, the counselor or therapist must keep the client's well-being front and center, both in the short term and the long term. If a client's ideological extremism seems to negatively affect mental health, relationships, and ability to function, this becomes an important focus of treatment. The therapist should help the client gain insight into these negative impacts and collaboratively explore healthier ways to channel and express their strongly held beliefs and values. Deviations from this norm are and should occur only in very unusual situations where others are likely to be imminently harmed.

The principle of **Autonomy**, which gained prominence in the late 20th century, is another ethical mandate (Raguram, 2016). Drawing on a tradition first elucidated by Immanuel Kant, this principle dictates that mental health professionals must respect a client's right to self-determination, even when the client's values and goals diverge significantly from those of the therapist. As we noted in earlier chapters, this is one of the hardest parts of working with a client with different political views than our own. A client who holds extreme political views is still entitled to chart their path in life as long as they are not infringing on the rights and freedoms of others.

As one counselor in the Midwest said, *"They have the freedom to believe all kinds of stupid stuff. And I have the professional obligation to allow them to believe stupid stuff if they wish."*

The therapist should be mindful of the power differential in the therapeutic relationship and take care not to impose their worldview on the client or pressure them to change their political ideology. Doing so would undermine the client's autonomy and likely provoke resistance rather than growth. This has been a recurrent theme of every chapter in this volume.

Autonomy can be paradoxical. Counselors and therapists face a logical inconsistency when they attempt to impose a Kantian-like universal imperative on their clients' actions, as this very act undermines the principle of autonomy itself. Autonomy, by its nature, resists being enforced. Furthermore, autonomy does not override other ethical imperatives. A therapist cannot remain a passive enabler if a client is engaging in behavior that is clearly harmful to themselves or others. In such situations, the therapist must find ways to influence the client to reconsider their choices or intervene if the risk of harm is imminent.

The principle of **Justice** has deep historical roots, which require that all clients be treated fairly and equitably, regardless of their ideological views (Hanlon, 2008). Extending from Biblical and Aristotelian traditions, it gained acceptance in the 20th century with the works of Rawls (1971), which emphasized justice as fairness. It is now accepted that a medical provider or therapist must offer the same quality of care and consideration to all clients or patients. As we have emphasized, for mental health providers, this can be challenging when a client expresses views that the therapist finds abhorrent or offensive.

For example, one of the authors recalled feeling utter frustration and revulsion during therapeutic interactions with a Civil War revisionist who suffered from depression. This client's seeming obsession with "The War of Northern Aggression" and positive remarks about chattel slavery, which were frequently brought up in therapy sessions, was particularly repugnant. However, these views had nothing to do with her ongoing depression, which had been triggered by loss and prolonged grief. In cases like this, a counselor or therapist must do the difficult internal work to manage their reactions and maintain a stance of openness, curiosity, and compassion for the client as a whole person. This does not mean agreeing with or absolving the client's ideology but rather extending to them the same basic human respect and dignity accorded to all people.

Fidelity refers to the mental health professional's duty to be truthful, keep promises, and uphold commitments to clients (Knapp & Fingerhut, 2024). The concept had roots in the Hippocratic Oath, but in mental health, was largely shaped by the contributions of Humanistic Psychologists stressing genuineness. When working with highly partisan clients, fidelity may require the therapist to have difficult but honest conversations about the limits of confidentiality and the boundaries of the therapeutic relationship.

For example, if a client discloses a credible plan to commit a violent hate crime based on their ideological extremism, there is no ethical dilemma. The mental health professional would have an ethical (and likely legal) duty to break confidentiality in order to warn and protect potential victims. The mental health professional should make these limits of confidentiality clear to partisan clients from the beginning while also emphasizing that their goal is to help the client, not to judge or punish them for their beliefs. The practice of reviewing the importance of and the limits to confidentiality should always be clearly agreed upon prior to beginning therapeutic work.

Fidelity also means following through on the treatment plan and therapeutic contract established with the client. If a therapist agrees to help an ideologically extreme client work on managing their anger or developing greater empathy for other perspectives, they need to attempt to follow through. In that case, it is incumbent on them to make a faithful effort to do so, even when the client's views create personal discomfort for the therapist. Terminating a client earlier than anticipated because of their political views is ethically questionable and would be justified only under extreme circumstances.

Ethical Practices with Partisan Clients

Ethical practices are founded on these key big five principles. Their operationalization encompasses many areas, including informed consent, confidentiality, and competence. Informed consent ensures that clients have sufficient information to make autonomous decisions about their treatment options (Knapp & Fingerhut, 2024). Confidentiality requires mental health professionals to protect client privacy except in specific, justified circumstances which primarily include duty to warn in cases of clear and immediate intention to commit murder or suicide and reporting information about the abuse or neglect of those in vulnerable populations; children, the elderly, and disabled persons. Competence necessitates ongoing professional development to maintain proficiency and effectively address client needs. All these principles can be more challenging to uphold when working with highly partisan clients.

Managing boundaries in counseling and therapy is another important practice intrinsically linked to the ethical principles of doing good (beneficence), doing no harm (non-maleficence), and protecting autonomy (Strohm Kitchener & Anderson, 2011). By maintaining clear boundaries, therapists create a safe and structured environment, the therapy space, that fosters the client's well-being and promotes positive therapeutic outcomes. Proper boundary management ensures that therapy remains client-centered, addressing specific needs and goals rather than being derailed by the therapist's personal biases or external issues. Additionally, clear boundaries prevent harmful interactions and maintain professionalism, protecting the client from emotional distress or psychological harm.

Effective boundary management also respects the client's right to make their own decisions and hold their own beliefs, even if these beliefs differ from the therapist's. It ensures that clients are fully informed and voluntarily consent to the therapeutic process, understanding their treatment options and the nature of the therapy. In this way, managing boundaries is essential for adhering to these ethical principles, ensuring that therapists act in the best interest of their clients, prevent harm, and respect their clients' autonomy, ultimately leading to more effective and ethical therapeutic practices.

Managing boundaries with a highly partisan therapy client can be challenging due to the strong emotional responses and intense political views involved. Therapists must maintain a neutral stance and avoid letting their personal beliefs influence the therapeutic process. Establishing and maintaining a therapeutic alliance can be difficult if the client perceives the therapist as opposing their political views. Clear boundaries and ground rules regarding political discussions are essential to keep the focus on the client's mental health needs rather than turning sessions into political debates. Throughout the volume we have emphasized that the mental health professional's political beliefs are not the focus of treatment. However, therapists and counselors must be honest about them, and then move on.

Cultural competence is a cornerstone of ethical practice (Parsonson, 2021). It involves understanding, respecting, and appropriately responding to the unique cultural backgrounds and belief systems of clients. A counselor or therapist who understands and respects these beliefs is better equipped to support clients in making informed choices about their treatment and their lives (Pearson, 2017). For politically partisan clients, this means acknowledging their political perspectives and ensuring that these views are considered in the therapeutic process. By doing so, the therapist empowers the client to take an active role in their therapy, making decisions that align with their values and beliefs. Cultural competence involves familiarity, although not a voyeuristic curiosity. Keeping this balance helps us support our clients effectively and respectfully.

> Working with clients from all sorts of backgrounds, I've seen that everyone views the world differently, whether they're accountants, sex workers, teachers, or artists. Good therapists need to get these different perspectives at least enough to listen and ask intelligent questions without letting their own beliefs get in the way. It's important to be curious and engaged, but not to ask questions just out of nosiness.
>
> *(Ron, a social worker in the Deep South)*

Professional integrity is another ethical practice. It emphasizes honesty, transparency, and ethical conduct in all professional interactions. This means that the decision to disclose and discuss the client's political beliefs must be made in the best interest of the client. Similarly, the disclosure of one's own biases and blind spots can be a significant challenge in therapeutic practice, particularly when working with highly partisan clients. If a client suspects that you have a different political perspective and raises that question, it's important to be honest and straightforward. They're probably asking out of concern for whether you can listen to them without judgment; whether you're trustworthy or not. The therapist can be curious about what brought the client's concern up during the session, but avoiding the question or reframing it as something else is likely to be met with increased concern by the client. An honest response might be:

> I appreciate your curiosity about my beliefs. While I may not agree with some of your thoughts or beliefs, that doesn't mean I don't respect and appreciate those differences. If you feel at any point that I'm judging you or reacting negatively to what you're sharing, I hope that you'll do what you just did: ask me and we'll talk about that.

While empirical data on this issue is limited, there is a growing concern that the current landscape of mental health practice may contribute to these blind spots. In today's fast-paced and high-demand environment, many counselors and therapists may not prioritize personal therapy and reflective practices as much as they should. This lack of attention to their own mental and emotional health can lead to unrecognized biases and blind spots that impact their professional work.

Without regular self-reflection and supervision, mental health professionals can become susceptible to letting their own political beliefs and biases influence their interactions with clients. This can be particularly problematic when working with clients who hold strong partisan views that differ from the therapist's own beliefs. The avoidance of personal therapy can result in a failure to address and mitigate these biases, leading to less effective and potentially harmful therapeutic interventions. Additionally, the emotional labor involved in working with highly polarized clients can be taxing, making it even more crucial for therapists to engage in regular self-care and reflective practices.

The increasing polarization in society means that therapists are more likely to encounter clients with extreme or strongly held political beliefs. This makes it imperative for mental health professionals to be vigilant about their own reactions and to strive for cultural competence and impartiality. Engaging in personal therapy can provide therapists with the tools to understand better and manage their own biases, ultimately leading to more effective and ethical practice.

Incorporating regular supervision, peer consultation, and personal therapy into a therapist's routine can help identify and address these behavioral blind spots (Terjesen & Del Vecchio, 2023). This commitment to ongoing personal and professional development not only benefits the therapist but also enhances the therapeutic experience for clients, fostering an environment where all clients feel respected and understood, regardless of their political beliefs.

Social responsibility is another ethical practice. For many professionals, it extends the ethical obligation beyond individuals, demanding that professionals advocate for mental health policies, address social determinants to mental health, and promote equity of access to care (Dyer, 2021). These principles collectively provide a comprehensive framework for ethical practice in mental health, ensuring that professionals uphold high standards of care, respect client autonomy, and contribute positively to both individual client outcomes and broader societal well-being.

Advocacy and Actions for Practitioners and the Mental Health Professions

As partisan polarization continues to intensify in society, it is increasingly important for mental health practitioners to be well-equipped to provide effective and ethical care to clients across the political spectrum. Advocacy for mental health practitioner training programs should prioritize cultural humility as a core competency. Curricula must emphasize the importance of approaching clients with openness, curiosity, and a willingness to step outside one's own ideological echo chamber. Assignments that encourage perspective-taking, such as conducting in-depth interviews with people who hold contrasting political views, are crucial for building this skill.

Practicing therapists should commit to examining their own assumptions and challenging themselves to consider issues from multiple angles. Instructors, supervisors, and colleagues must encourage therapists to read a diverse array of news sources, engage in respectful dialogue with those who disagree, and be vigilant against resorting to stereotyping. This will help them embody cultural humility in their work with ideologically diverse clients.

Beyond this, we propose that we include political ideology in discussions of intersectionality. Cultural competency training often highlights intersectionality, recognizing that individuals hold multiple intersecting identities shaping their experiences and worldviews. However, political affiliation and ideology are frequently overlooked as important intersectional factors. Advocacy efforts should push for graduate programs and continuing education training to explicitly include political diversity alongside other elements of identity. Practitioners must be prompted to reflect on how a client's ideology may interact with their race, gender, religion, sexual orientation, disability status, and other personal characteristics and values. Including training in political diversity is necessary to develop more holistic conceptualizations and treatment plans.

Advocacy is also needed to ensure practitioners develop concrete skills for engaging in respectful dialogue with clients holding different political views. Training in communication techniques such as active listening, motivational interviewing, Socratic questioning, and I-statements should be prioritized to navigate the unique challenges of political discussions. Role-playing exercises where trainees practice having difficult conversations related to partisan issues can boost practitioner confidence and competence. Supervisors should be encouraged to model and coach supervisees through challenging moments of political dialogue with clients as they arise.

Advocates must also highlight the importance of training practitioners to tolerate and work with inevitable value discrepancies, especially in today's politically polarized climate. Training should normalize the experience of value conflicts and provide frameworks for resolving them ethically. Student trainees and practitioners need guidance in distinguishing between situations where value differences can be bracketed for the client's benefit and those presenting a true ethical impasse. Advocacy efforts should push for trainees to deeply consider their personal "red lines" and develop scripts for addressing these issues tactfully.

Mental health professionals must also be encouraged to explore their potential biases and blind spots related to political ideology, just as they do with other domains of identity. Advocacy should focus on guiding educators and supervisors to help practitioners examine how their upbringing, social context, moral foundations, and life experiences have shaped their ideological instincts and political identities. Therapists who see themselves as a "blank slate" regarding politics and related social issues are not well prepared to work with political differences in their clients. As we noted in Chapter 11, training in depolarization can build a better sense of how to respond and react to those with different worldviews.

Reflecting on "hot button" partisan issues and considering their impact on interactions with clients can enhance self-awareness. Tools like ideological autobiographies, implicit bias assessments with a political focus, and candid peer discussions can aid practitioners in recognizing their biases more clearly. When roll-playing with other students in clinical training, issues related to politics and social issues can help trainees develop necessary skills for working with politically diverse clients and help identify values or beliefs that may be difficult for them to address therapeutically.

Advocacy is also necessary to make practitioners aware of how they may unwittingly communicate their political affiliations through subtle choices like office décor, reading materials, or casual comments. While perfect political neutrality is impossible, practitioners should critically examine their environment and interactions for unintended partisan signaling. What magazines are in the waiting room? Art or books that are in the office space? For example, the use of identifying pronouns (she/her, they/them) are likely to signal a liberal orientation to more conservative clients.

When political self-disclosures occur, therapists should process them with clients and assess their impact on the therapeutic relationship. Supervisors can help supervisees practice reorienting conversations back to the client's experience and treatment goals. How to get a session back on track when there's been a disconnect is an important skill as a therapist.

Advocates should also emphasize the importance of identifying and validating the strengths within clients' ideological worldviews. All belief systems, even those that may seem rigid or misguided, develop for compelling and self-protective reasons.

Educators are encouraged to assign readings that highlight the psychological functions and moral underpinnings of both liberal and conservative belief systems. Trainees must practice extracting the "kernel of truth" from opposing political talking points and reflecting it back in an affirming way. This is an important part of therapist training in diversity similar to learning about histories of oppression with different populations.

Advocates must also recognize that conservative clients, particularly those from rural areas, may face distinct barriers to feeling understood and accepted in therapy. Practitioners are encouraged to make services accessible and welcoming to traditionally underserved conservative populations by offering telehealth sessions, sliding scale fees, and advertising in venues frequented by right-leaning individuals.

Liberal leaning therapists should be educated about the values, traditions, and beliefs common in local conservative communities. Conservative therapists can do the same with liberal ideology and history. When worldview differences arise in treatment, therapists must manage their reactions skillfully to keep the client engaged. It's helpful to have some understanding of the history and values of the other side's perspective to assure client's feel respected and appreciated.

Mental health practitioners have a responsibility to advocate for strong and clear ethical standards, ensuring services are accessible to all clients, regardless of race, class, location, religion, or political orientation. Advocacy should focus on engaging students in discussions of how core ethical principles like beneficence, non-maleficence, justice, autonomy, and fidelity apply uniquely when working with conservative and liberal clients.

Professional organizations must continue to promulgate clear ethical guidelines around political diversity, and graduate programs should integrate these guidelines into training and supervision. By advocating for a strong shared ethical foundation, the mental health field can create a culture committed to providing all clients with high-quality and culturally responsive care. Educators, supervisors, and leaders in the profession have a special responsibility to champion these ethical values for the new generation of practitioners.

The Bigger Picture

Our professions are currently undergoing another shift that is widening our scope beyond family relationships and exploring the context of our social, ideological, and political histories. It's become important to understand the influence and impact of our race, ethnicity, sexual orientation, gender identification, religious/ spiritual beliefs, generational history, and other factors that define our lives, including our political beliefs. We are more than individuals, more than family members; we are part of a larger network of ideologies, histories, influences, affiliations, social groups, and institutions. All of these play an important role in our sense of self and our mental and emotional well-being. Our professions can play a vital role in being of service to not only our students and clients but also our neighborhoods, communities, and country.

As the mental health profession has expanded, many of us have become more interested in working beyond our offices to serve others. Some of our professions, like Social Work and Human Services, have a foundational focus on not just individuals, but the context of their lives. In those disciplines, workplaces are more likely to be community based and focused on how to best serve certain populations rather than being primarily focused on the medical model of serving individuals who are experiencing behavioral, emotional, or neurological disorders. For many of us, such as licensed professional counselors (LPC's), licensed marriage and family therapists (LMFT's), and psychologists

(PhD, PsyD, and EdD's), much of our training continues to follow the model of focusing on the internal life of an individual or on specific relationship problems within a family or couple.

When the field of family therapy developed in the 1960–1970s, it was the beginning of seeing the individual client in the context of their relationships (Suppes, 2023). An appreciation of how clients were impacted by family and intimate partnerships offered us a very different perspective on many of the "disorders" that we were treating. It was an intuitive understanding of how important those relationship experiences were in our development and overall mental well-being that led to the expansion of our focus. The historical impact of family relationships, as reported by individual clients, only gave us one perspective. That changed when we began bringing in other family members and could directly observe how patterns of interaction, roles in the family, alliances between family members, and numerous other factors came into play in client's lives. A better understanding of family influences and dynamics gave us a much more complex and comprehensive understanding of the problems or issues that brought clients to therapy.

The book "We've Had a Hundred Years of Psychotherapy—and the World's Getting Worse" (1993) by James Hillman, a Jungian psychologist, and Michael Ventura, a journalist, was a call to examine a professional role beyond the confines of an office. The book described how psychotherapists viewed human dilemmas as an internal, personal problem, somehow disconnected from the world we inhabit. The authors envisioned a psychology that incorporated the context in which a person lives; the social and political forces that impacted both our physical and mental well-being. They proposed that "… therapy, in it's crazy way, by emphasizing the inner soul and ignoring the outer soul, supports the decline of the actual world" (p. 5). At the time, this was a startling idea; that psychotherapy could further open the door to work with people in the context of their culture, community, and world. More importantly, not only could we incorporate these public aspects of our lives into our work, but it was important that we do so for the betterment of the world.

How are we impacted psychologically and emotionally by social change, politics, economics, and all the other factors and forces that affect us? Is there a place in psychotherapy to address the pain and challenges that are part of being in the world? Might our pursuit of helping others include encouraging them to be engaged citizens who participate in causes that are important to them? Finally, might we, as mental health providers do the same and devote some of our time and effort to improving the conditions in which both we and our clients reside? The American Mental Health Counselors Association (AMHCA), American Counseling Association (ACA), National Organization for Human Services (NOHS), and National Association of Social Workers (NASW) have sections in their ethics codes that encourage us to advocate at institutional and societal levels to foster sociopolitical change and address potential obstacles that impact the welfare of our clients (Whalen, 2023).

The challenge to MHP's is how to incorporate these factors into the work that we do. We're expanding our perspective to create a better understanding of the individual through a deeper and more complete awareness of how they are responding to those forces in their lives that are either helpful or detrimental to them. Especially in this time of political polarization, mental health professionals can play a larger role in enhancing our ability to communicate and connect to people with whom we don't always agree. We can participate more fully in discussions beyond those focused on the well-being of individuals and find ways to influence the context in which we all live. We can bring our expertise, based on research and clinical experience, to improve the functioning of our society and politics.

Public Trust

For many people, there are huge "red flags" around mental health professionals weighing in on social and political issues. There's been a growing distrust of science in general, and psychological research in particular, on the part of a significant number of our citizens. Psychotherapists are often seen as "elitists" or authoritarians, and there is justifiable concern about the history of discrimination and abuses that have been part of our field. We have made mistakes and done harm. Research like the Stanford Prison Experiment (Zimbardo, Haney, Banks, & Joffe, 1971) and the clinical practice of Rebirthing Therapy (Josefson, 2001) are examples of mistakes that were made with human subjects and clients. We believe, however, that the professions have responded to those mistakes by building stronger ethical codes, emphasizing training in ethical research and clinical practices and procedures, developing more evidence-based foundations for clinical approaches, incorporating cultural awareness courses in our curricula, and inviting greater public scrutiny of our methods and practices.

An important aspect to consider when determining whether to become more active in social and political issues is humility. Regardless of the rigor and breadth of research in our field, we don't have all the answers. Science, particularly the social sciences, is not a perfect approach to understanding ourselves and our world. A student in one of the author's "Introduction to Psychology" class once asked "How much can you trust a science that's largely based on experiments with college sophomores and white rats?" Don't expect everyone to accept what you share or believe that your information is valid or valuable. Offer what you have to offer with humility and accept questions and criticisms with grace and an open mind. Often, our students, clients, and members of the public see the negative impact of our work before it's clear to us. Acknowledge that we don't know everything about those topics that we research and keep an open mind about what other perspectives, like religious beliefs or cultural traditions have to offer. Importantly, be informed about the arguments that are likely to be made countering what you believe. Seek out information or have conversations with those who have a different perspective than yours. Challenge yourself to see the issue from another viewpoint.

What Is a "Citizen Therapist"?

Historically, our professional training and ethics codes have cautioned us to avoid moving beyond our role as consultants to individuals suffering from defined mental, emotional, neurological or relationship difficulties. Mental health professionals often play a limited role in addressing societal and political issues that have a detrimental influence on individuals, their families, and our communities. "What can we do in the face of poverty, disease, war, injustice, and environmental devastation … Our psychologies tend to treat this as a personal problem, but it is not" (Kornfield, 2008, p. 353). All of us suffer from the effects of these problems, whether personally or through our awareness of the suffering of others. We are impacted by both our own and other's experiences through the preponderance of images and stories that pour in through news and social media. "This is a pressing problem for psychology" (Kornfield, 2008, p. 353). We can enlarge our role and contribute to making a more compassionate and safer world for all of us to inhabit.

In his book, "The Ethical Lives of Clients: Transcending Self-Interest in Psychotherapy" (2022) Dr. William Doherty introduced the term "citizen therapist." He argued for therapists to become more "… skilled, sensitive, and intentional about addressing ethical issues in therapy" so that we can not only help a client with specific personal issues but also work with them to contribute to "… building a more connected and just world" (p. 15). He developed this concept to encourage MHP's who are interested in working with the "personal and public worlds of clients and being willing to engage directly in promoting the health of communities and the larger world" (p. 131) to engage as a citizen therapist. This perspective expands the potential impact we can have in our professional roles. The citizen therapist is one who is active in their community and/or country to address the social and political forces that impact the emotional and mental well-being of everyone.

The citizen therapist perspective is more clearly described in the recent book, "Becoming a Citizen Therapist" (Doherty & Mendenhall, 2024). They envision a more public role for therapists who want to offer their expertise to help people "… connect to their communities and solve social problems" (p. 4). The work of the citizen therapist is to unite with other citizens to organize and take responsibility for their communities and identify projects that can create needed changes. We provide our expertise in helping community members from diverse political, social, economic, and other perspectives to work together to solve problems. It's something we know how to do. It's also what is needed to maintain and strengthen a democracy; "… 'we the diverse people' taking responsibility for solving our collective problems" (p. 13).

The citizen therapist model invites us to partner with diverse representatives, coalitions, and other interested citizens with a focus on collective, transformative action. Our role is to bring the knowledge and skills we embody in our professions to address ongoing concerns such as climate change, addiction, disenfranchisement, healthcare, education, and social assistance programs; those issues that are best addressed by both government and communities working together. Doherty and Mendenhall (2024) describe these aspects of being a citizen therapist:

Being a citizen therapist incorporates:

- An identity as a citizen with professional skills and expertise working with other citizen experts to solve community problems.
- An understanding of how society and culture can negatively impact people and create or enhance conditions that contribute to mental health problems such as isolation, stigmatization, violence, and depression.
- A set of skills for assisting people in coming together to connect and engage in public education and action to meet community needs (pp. 25–26).
- Assisting in research on the effectiveness of programs and projects to maximize their effectiveness and address negative outcomes.

This model stresses the importance of civic engagement to strengthen personal health and social well-being, the need to transcend the traditional provider-consumer model of health care … and a vision of ordinary citizens creating initiatives in partnership with therapists and other professionals.

(p. 27)

There are different aspects of being a citizen therapist that we can assume. All of these are cooperative, consulting roles and not a "top down" approach in which we assume control of the work. Doherty and Mendenhall (2024) describe three important roles we can take on: educator, advocate, and organizer. An educator is someone who brings important resources to the community. They share information, consultation, and skills that might be needed to enhance the knowledge that exists already in the community. Advocates collaborate with those in the community who are working for change through influencing policymakers. They may assist with educational efforts on topics of interest to the community and to political representatives. Organizers are "… conveners, facilitators, and process leaders" for community interests and projects. They partner with groups who are interested in change and offer both professional knowledge and skills in working with relationships and groups.

How We Can Make a Difference

The following are two examples of issues that citizen therapists could connect with others to address. It's important to emphasize that these activities are not designed by MHP's and forced on the community, they are resources and actions designed in cooperation with community members. The possibilities are limitless; there's a place for any MHP who's interested in being a citizen therapist to have a role in supporting social change.

Reducing Anger and Hostility

Political polarization is one of the forces at work in the United States and many other nations that has created distress for so many of us. One important goal in writing this book is to enhance our understanding of the emotional and psychological impact of extreme partisanship and how MHP's can incorporate information and skills to help all of us effectively cope with this phenomenon. Many of us, regardless of our political affiliation, have concerns that our democracy may be broken or failing. Certainly, most of us are affected by the level of anger and animosity that emerges when certain topics are raised. In the book "American Rage: How Anger Shapes Our Politics" (Weber, 2020), the author focuses on the shift in our political discourse in which we're more governed by the bonds of negativity toward our political enemies than by a positive attachment to our preferred political party. While some people on both sides of the political spectrum may dislike some of their party's representatives, they would never vote across political lines. We increasingly tend to vote "the party" and not the individual.

As mental health professionals we understand the corrosive impact of prolonged rage; that it becomes a poison we drink hoping the other person will die. Staicu and Cuţov (2010, November 15) reported a positive correlation between prolonged, high levels of anger and Type 2 diabetes, coronary disease, bulimia, and dangerous driving (road rage). They concluded that

> Because the scientific literature demonstrated the connection between anger, hostility and aggressiveness and various health risks, the intervention for healing or preventing these diseases should not only be pharmacological, but also psychological; therapists should insist on ways of managing these behaviors in order to prevent diseases and any kind of risk that they could involve.
>
> *(p. 374)*

We would add that this doesn't have to be a "one person at a time" endeavor; it is an issue that affects communities, and we can address anger problems at that level. While excessive anger itself is not a mental disorder, it certainly has a negative impact on not only the person expressing it but also family and social relationships. Citizens in democracies have always disagreed passionately about social issues and we always will; the problem is the level of contempt that we express toward each other. In addition to depolarizing, we must also learn and help others to de-escalate, often one person at a time.

As a citizen therapist, some of the ways we can help are to:

- Intervene when those we agree with politically exhibit contempt for the other side. It's important that we let our family, friends, students, colleagues, and others know that we pledge to refrain from demeaning, disrespectful, angry commentary about those with whom we disagree. We can invite them to do so as well.
- Practice and promote de-escalation and anger management. We train ourselves and practice engaging peacefully and respectfully with others in our therapy space, the classroom, at conferences or trainings, and wherever else we might have the opportunity to assist others in finding calm connections amid the chaos.
- Create programs or training with community partners based on well-established anger management techniques such as active listening and self-regulation.

Identifying Misinformation

The American Psychological Association (APA, 2023) has been focusing efforts on how to identify and intervene in the spread of disinformation, especially as it relates to healthcare. In the COVID epidemic, many of us had clients, friends, and family members who were unsure of what to believe about the nature of the illness and what precautions to take. Many of us worked with clients and students who came to distrust long established and highly regarded sources of health information like the Center for Disease Control (CDC) in favor of both political and medical leaders who opposed some of the recommendations such as wearing masks and closing schools to limit the spread of the disease. People began to divide into oppositional groups depending on their sources of information. Misinformation proliferated, such as the idea that there were "tracking devices" implanted in the vaccines. The closing of schools was a decision that many disagreed with and that has had significant negative repercussions for many children. We didn't know who to trust and our communities and the country became increasingly divided over how to respond to this challenge.

It's almost certain that we'll face more of this type of challenge in the future as we experience outbreaks of other diseases and illnesses. Our professions have an important role to play in combating falsehoods and rumors. As MHP's, we can help citizens, organizations, and the media to identify and confront misinformation. The APA (2023) report focused on the following questions:

- What are the psychological factors that make people susceptible to believe and act on misinformation?
- How and why does misinformation spread?
- What interventions can be used to counter misinformation effectively?

The report's recommendations encourage MHPs to collaborate with policymakers, community leaders, the public, and the media to address the ongoing risk of misinformation to health, well-being (both physical and psychological), and civic life.

As (Doherty & Mendenhall, 2024) have noted, as citizen therapists some of the ways we can help are to:

- Avoid repeating misinformation without including a correction.
- Collaborate with social media companies to understand and reduce the spread of harmful misinformation.
- Use misinformation correction strategies with tools already proven to promote healthy behaviors (e.g., counseling, skills training, incentives, social norms).
- Leverage trusted sources to counter misinformation and provide accurate health information.
- Debunk misinformation often and repeatedly using evidence-based methods.
- Prebunk misinformation to inoculate susceptible audiences by building skills and resilience from an early age.
- Demand data access and transparency from social media companies for scientific research on misinformation.
- Fund basic and translational research into the psychology of health misinformation, including effective ways to counter it (American Psychological Association, 2024).

To reiterate, becoming more active professionally outside of our clinics and offices is not for everyone. However, for those who want to contribute on a public level and devote time to share their skills as mental health professionals, we encourage exploration and collaboration in whatever way fits with your interests and skills. We can bring an important perspective to the public square.

Summary

As this chapter has outlined, there are many concrete actions mental health practitioners and educators can take to promote competence in the field. From emphasizing cultural humility and dialogue skills in graduate training, to encouraging ideological self-awareness in clinical practice, to upholding clear ethical standards in partisan work, there are transformative opportunities at both the individual and institutional level.

Pursuing these opportunities is both an ethical mandate and a clinical necessity in our current political climate. As partisan tensions fuel increasing rates of emotional distress, relationship conflict, and other mental health concerns, any therapist who serves the public must be prepared to work skillfully with conservative and liberal worldviews alike.

By embracing the recommendations outlined here with openness, humility and conviction, mental health practitioners can rise to the challenge of providing care across the partisan divide. In so doing, we reaffirm our professional commitment to understanding and serving all those who seek our support, regardless of ideological differences. This is the heart of ethical and effective practice. It will become more important in the coming years.

References

American Psychological Association (March 1, 2024). *8 recommendations for countering misinformation: Specific ways to meet the ongoing risk of misinformation to health, well-being, and civic life.* Retrieved from: www.apa.org/topics/journalism-facts/mis information-recommendations

Doherty, W. J. (2022). *The ethical lives of clients: Transcending self-interest in psychotherapy.* Washington, DC: American Psychological Association.

Doherty, W. J., & Mendenhall, T. J. (2024). *Becoming a citizen therapist: Integrating community problem-solving into your work as a healer.* Washington, DC: American Psychological Association.

Dyer, A. R., Kohrt, B. A., & Candilis, P. J. (2021). *Global Mental Health Ethics.* New York: Springer International Publishing. https://hsrc.himmelfarb.gwu.edu/books/269

Hanlon, C. R. (2008). Ethical principles for everyone in health care. In S. W. A. Gunn & M. Masellis (Eds.), *Concepts and practice of humanitarian medicine* (pp. 67–77). New York, NY: Springer Science + Business Media.

Hillman, J., & Ventura, M. (1993). *We've had a hundred years of psychotherapy – And the world's getting worse.* New York, NY: Harper Collins.

Josefson, D. (2001, April 28). Rebirthing therapy banned after girl died in 70 minute struggle. *BMJ, 322*(7293), 1014. PMCID: PMC1174742.

Knapp, S. J., & Fingerhut, R. (2024). *Practical ethics for psychologists: A positive approach* (4th ed.). Washington, DC: American Psychological Association.

Kornfield, J. (2008). *The wise heart: A guide to the universal teachings of Buddhist psychology.* New York, NY: Bantam Books.

Mishna, F., Underwood, M. K., Milne, C., & Gibson, M. F. (2013). Ethical issues. In S. Bauman, D. Cross, & J. Walker (Eds.), *Principles of cyberbullying research: Definitions, measures, and methodology* (pp. 148–165). Oxford: Routledge.

Parsonson, K. L. (2021). The universal declaration of ethical principles for psychologists. In K. L. Parsonson (Ed.), *Handbook of international psychology ethics: Codes and commentary from around the world* (pp. 240–243). London: Routledge/Taylor & Francis Group.

Pearson, G. S. (2017). Culture and cultural dilemmas. In D. B. Cooper (Ed.), *Ethics in mental health-substance use* (pp. 86–98). London: Routledge/Taylor & Francis Group.

Raguram, R. (2016). Ethics in therapeutic practice: Culturally universal and valid? In P. Bhola & A. Raguram (Eds.), *Ethical issues in counselling and psychotherapy practice: Walking the line* (pp. 187–197). New York: Springer Science + Business Media. https://doi.org/10.1007/978-981-10-1808-4_12

Rawls, J. (1971). *A theory of justice.* Boston: Harvard College. ISBN 0-674-01772-2.

Staicu, M. L., & Cuțov, M. (2010) Anger and health risk behaviors. *Journal of Medicine and Life*, *3*(4), 372–375. PMID: 21254733; PMCID: PMC3019061. www.ncbi.nlm.nih.gov/pmc/articles/PMC3019061/

Strohm Kitchener, K., & Anderson, S. K. (2011). *Foundations of ethical practice, research, and teaching in psychology and counseling* (2nd ed.). London: Routledge/Taylor & Francis Group.

Suppes, B. C. (2023). *Family systems theory simplified: Applying and understanding systemic therapy models.* New York, NY: Taylor and Francis.

Terjesen, M. D., & Del Vecchio, T. (2023). *Handbook of training and supervision in cognitive behavioral therapy.* Springer Nature Switzerland.

Weber, S. W. (August 27, 2020). *American rage: How anger shapes our politics.* Cambridge: Cambridge University Press.

Whalen, M. E. (2023). *Ethical considerations for therapists in the age of climate emergency.* Resources/Ethical-Consideration-for-Therapists-in-the-Climate-Emergency-Michael-Whalen-9-01-20.pdf

Zimbardo, P. G., Haney, C., Banks, W. C., & Jaffe, D. (1974). The psychology of imprisonment: Privation, power and pathology. In Z. Rubin (Ed.), *Doing unto others: Explorations in social behavior* (pp. 61–73). Englewood Cliffs, NJ: Prentice-Hall.

APPENDIX A

Political Orientation and Therapeutic Outcomes[1]

Our ongoing research (Keiser & McCown, submitted) examines the intersection of political orientation and therapeutic outcomes. We administered a computerized version of Everett's (2013) 12-item Social and Economic Conservatism Scale (SECS) to 645 counselors and therapists (413 women) over a four-year period. The SECS is a self-report measure designed to assess political orientation across two dimensions: social and economic conservatism. It is particularly useful because it measures people's support for aspects of conservatism regardless of party affiliation or self-identified designation as being Right or Left. Each of the 12 questions was initially scored on a 100-point distribution but transformed for reporting on a scale from 0 to 10, where 0 represents the most progressive values and 10 represents the most conservative. The distribution of all data was approximately normal.

Along with SECS scores, we collected demographic data, including gender, geographic location, theoretical orientation, and professional affiliation or training. Theoretical orientations were rated on a 100-point scale across seven categories: psychodynamic/psychoanalytic, behavioral/cognitive behavioral/cognitive, systemic, feminist, multicultural, humanistic/existentialist, and biological/neurobehavioral. The results revealed that mental health professionals, on average, hold political values more closely aligned with Democrats or Independents based on a comparison with the norms from Everett's findings. The mean SECS score for the therapist group, transformed to the 0 to 10 scale, was 4.80 (SD = 2.76), indicating moderate liberalism.

No significant geographic differences were observed across the five regions (Northeast, South, Midwest, Mountains, and West Coast), which was surprising. One possible explanation is that the study's geographic categorization may have grouped together regions that, despite geographic proximity, have distinct cultural, social, or political attitudes. By lumping disparate regions into broader categories, the instrument may have obscured meaningful regional differences, thereby attenuating any potential findings. Among professional affiliations, social workers were found to be the most politically liberal, followed by psychologists, physicians/nurses, and finally, professional counselors, who were the least progressive.

However, only the difference between social workers and professional counselors reached statistical significance. No gender differences emerged, which contradicts previous research suggesting that women tend to lean more progressive. Additionally, no clear relationship was found between theoretical orientation and political values, likely due to difficulties in accurately measuring theoretical constructs. Differences among people of color and sexual minorities would be interesting to explore but were not included in this study.

In the second part of this study, we surveyed 212 former psychotherapy clients (139 women) regarding their political orientations and therapeutic experiences. The average SECS score for this group, also transformed to the 0 to 10 scale, was 7.44 (SD = 2.91), indicating a more conservative alignment compared to the therapists. Clients were also asked to compare their political views with those of their therapists on the same scale, and on average, clients rated themselves as 2.1 points more conservative than their therapists. Clients further rated the effectiveness of therapy on a 100-point scale for how much they felt the therapy helped them, which was also transformed to fit the 0 to 10 scale. Unsurprisingly, clients who perceived their therapist as more politically progressive than themselves rated the therapy as less effective. The strongest predictor of high therapy ratings was the congruence between the client's values and their perception of the therapist's values, with a correlation of $r = .31$, a statistically significant effect. Therapist gender and age differences were not significant predictors of self-reported therapy value.

A smaller number (N-37) of clients rated their therapists as more conservative than themselves. These people also had a poor self-reported outcome. Thirteen of these people (35%) terminated treatment in two or fewer sessions. While there are many possible reasons for this, including diagnostic factors, this finding needs further research.

Regardless, these preliminary findings are significant because they suggest that therapists and counselors may be perceived as having a negative impact on both conservative and liberal clients, mainly when there is a noticeable political incongruence between therapist and client. The study's results indicate that clients who see their therapists as more politically progressive tend to rate their therapeutic experiences less favorably. Those that see their therapists as less liberal than themselves also experience problems. Although retrospective accounts are fraught with theoretical concerns that may threaten valid conclusions, these findings are still worthy of reflection.

Note

1 We appreciate comments regarding data analysis and interpretation by several colleagues. Details regarding the ongoing study are available from at wgmccown1@ gmail.com.

APPENDIX B

Resources and Recommended Reading

These are highly recommended books that explore the political divide from a variety of perspectives. Our hope is that these resources will serve as starting points for your exploration and professional education in working across the political divide.

- Doherty, W. J. (2022). *The ethical lives of clients: Transcending self-interest in psychotherapy*. Washington, DC: American Psychological Association.
  - In this book, Doherty introduces the concept of a "citizen therapist" and advocates for expanding psychotherapy from an "individualist focus toward a more relational one" that includes addressing larger societal issues such as political polarization.
- Doherty, W. J., & Mendenhall, T. J. (2024). *Becoming a citizen therapist: Integrating community problem-solving into your work as a healer.* Washington, DC: American Psychological Association.
  - Doherty and Mendenhall's recent book expands on the concept of a "citizen therapist" and introduces the "citizen health care model" which incorporates community leaders and advocates to address health and mental wellness through development of local resources.
- Frisby, C. L., Redding, R. E., O'Donohue, W. T., & Lilienfeld, S.O. (Eds.) (2023). *Ideological and political bias in psychology: Nature, scope and solutions.* Cham, Switzerland: Springer.
  - This book (just under 1,000 pages) is a deep dive into examining assumptions and biases in both academia and professional practice in the mental health field. It's a contributed volume that offers a variety of perspectives for minimizing political influence in the training, research, and the practice of psychotherapy and counseling.

- Guzman, M. (2022). *I never thought of it that way: How to have fearlessly curious conversations in dangerously divided times*. Dallas, TX: BenBella Books, Inc.
  - A wonderful book on using "radical curiosity" to create connections between people with diverse beliefs.
- Haidt, J. (2012). *The righteous mind: Why good people are divided by politics and religion*. New York: Vintage Books.
  - Haidt's book is a "must read" for those who want to understand the moral foundations of political beliefs and how to better understand both liberal and conservative viewpoints. He also provides guidance for building connections across the ideological divide based on understanding and appreciation of both ideologies.
- Hibbing, J. R., Smith, K. B., & Alford, J. R. (2014*). Predisposed: Liberals, conservatives, and the biology of political differences*. New York: Routledge.
  - The authors explore the question of whether we are "hardwired" to be either liberal or conservative. They propose that our biology is a significant factor in predisposing us to see and understand the world in different ways and that these differences influence our political and ideological views. It's a fascinating, funny, thoughtful book for those interested in how we come to believe what we believe.
- Hillman, J., & Ventura, M. (1993). *We've had a hundred years of psychotherapy – And the world's getting worse*. New York: Harper Collins.
  - Hillman (a psychotherapist) and Ventura (a journalist) wrote this book from conversations they had exploring the foundation and purpose of psychotherapy. They questioned whether psychotherapists' responsibilities should extend beyond their clients to the wider public interest and whether psychotherapy could contribute to building a more just and compassionate world. Their conversation remains relevant today.
- Klein, E. (2020). *Why we're polarized*. New York: Avid Reader Press.
  - Klein is a journalist who traces the history of political polarization in the United States, particularly over the past several decades. He provides a map to understand how we've become so polarized and what steps we can take to better manage our political differences. (PLEASE NOTE THE CORRECT INFORMATION FOR RIPLEY AND INCLUDE HERE) lead to high conflict and how to help people break free of those patterns. It's a useful book in confronting our own conflict patterns and a guide to helping our clients.
- Safer, J. (2019). *I love you, but I hate your politics: How to protect your intimate relationships in a poisonous partisan world*. London: Biteback Publishing.
  - Safer is an experienced psychotherapist who works with couples and families impacted by political polarization. Her book is filled with case studies and guidelines on how to work with relationships affected

by contentious political differences. It's an important book for family therapists or for anyone confronting polarization in a relationship.

Resources for Information, Engagement, Training, and Support

When political or social issues arise in the therapy space, how can we continue to improve our knowledge and skills to establish and maintain an effective therapeutic relationship? Fortunately, there are organizations, workshops, discussion groups, and other resources that can help us depolarize and be more informed about working with polarized clients so that we can effectively connect to those across the political divide. For mental health professions to remain relevant and respected, we must commit to welcoming people from across the spectrum of political beliefs into the therapy space.

As mental health professionals we have a commitment to seek out research, information, and connection with teaching or training resources when developing new skills or working with unfamiliar issues or populations. The resources provided are all established, well-respected, and readily available to those who want to learn how to bridge the political divide. From our own experience, we know it can be challenging to open ourselves to encounters with people with whom we disagree. We all agree, however, that it's benefitted us personally and professionally and helped us be better citizens and therapists. We hope you'll experience that as well when you engage with and learn from others who are on that path. Many of these organizations and resources are also useful for students, trainees, and clients who are interested in their services.

Organizations:

- **Braver Angels**: Braver Angels was founded by a conservative and a liberal after the 2016 presidential election. The mission of Braver Angels is to "Bring Americans together to bridge the partisan divide and strengthen our democratic republic." Braver Angels is a non-profit volunteer organization dedicated to political depolarization and active engagement across ideologies. The organization offers workshops, debates, and other events where "red" (conservative) and "blue" (liberal) participants attempt to better understand one another's positions and discover their shared values. They provide both on-line and in person trainings, workshops, meetings, and other events across the country. Braver Angels is also a useful resource for clients and students.
  Contact: For more information: https://braverangels.org/

- **The Open Therapy Institute**: In an increasingly politicized culture, the Open Therapy Institute is helping therapists and clients, especially those who lean conservative, to find their voice, get support, and connect to others. The Institute is at the forefront of developing innovative, evidence-based tools to help therapy clients, train and support mental health clinicians, and address social issues.

The OTI provides resources for therapists through a variety of accredited training workshops (see "Workshops and Trainings"), research opportunities, and client referrals to approved members.

Contact: www.opentherapyinstitute.org/about

- **StoryCorps "One Small Step"**: StoryCorps is committed to the idea that everyone has an important story to tell and that everyone's story matters. The StoryCorps mission is to help us believe in each other by illuminating the humanity and possibility in us all—one story at a time. StoryCorps was founded in 2003 and has helped more than 640,000 people across the country have meaningful conversations about their lives. These recordings are collected in the U.S. Library of Congress and in an online archive which is now the largest single collection of human voices ever gathered. Created by StoryCorps, One Small Step is an effort to remind the country of the humanity in all of us, even those with whom we disagree. The initiative brings strangers with different political views together to record a 50-minute conversation— not to debate politics, but to learn who we are as people. Audio recordings of each interview are archived at the Library of Congress. Anyone can apply to be matched with a conversation partner. This is also a useful resource for clients and students.

    Contact: For more information: https://storycorps.org/discover/onesm all step/

- **Starts With Us**: Starts With Us is a growing movement with the mission of equipping Americans to overcome toxic polarization and effectively solve our toughest problems. Starts With Us uses media and technology to foster independent thinking and constructive communication across our differences, inspiring and empowering us to practice curiosity, compassion, and courage. Their website also offers a questionnaire to assess your level of polarization. This resource is useful with students and clients.

    Contact: For more information: startswith.us

Workshops and Trainings:

- **Braver Angels Workshops:** Braver Angels offers workshops on a regular basis free of charge (donations are requested but not required). There are three Beginner Workshops which are "Depolarizing Within," "Skills for Bridging the Divide," and "Skills for Social Media." The workshops are on-line group sessions that are focused on providing information and developing skills. They also offer training for "Families and Politics" to help develop skills for communicating with family members holding different political views. This is a very useful resource for clients and students as well as mental health professionals.

Contact: For more information: https://braverangels.org/attend-a-workshop/

- **The Open Therapy Institute:** The OTI offers a wide variety of accredited, on-line training workshops for mental health professionals. Workshop titles include: "Bias in Therapy," "Self-Censorship," "Overlooked Cultural Issues," and Racial/Cultural Reductionism." New workshops are constantly being developed and offered through the OTI which makes it a valuable resource for those of us, especially who are left leaning, to learn important skills in working effectively across the political gap.

  Contact: For more information: www.opentherapyinstitute.org/workshops-memberships

- **Bridging the Divide: Developing Relationships Between People with Diverse Views:** This on-line, 6-hour workshop is presented regularly by Cheryl Dolinger Brown, LCSW. It is an interactive workshop designed specifically for mental health professionals and there is a fee for participants. Six Continuing Education Units (CEU'S) are awarded on completion.

  Contact: For more information: cheryldolingerbrown.com

- **The Polarization Detox Challenge:** The Polarization Detox Challenge was developed by the Morton Deutsch International Center for Cooperation and Conflict Resolution at Columbia University, and the nonprofit Starts With Us. The Challenge is a free, online bootcamp supporting Americans in engaging in constructive conflict across differences and breaking free from toxic polarization. Once registered, participants have a daily challenge to assist in depolarizing. It's based on the book *The Way Out: How to Overcome Toxic Polarization* by Professor Peter T. Coleman.

  This training is also a useful resource for clients and students.

  Contact: For more information: https://startswith.us/pdc/?utm_source=Sto ryCorps+Email+Audience&utm_campaign=f15e7d2ea1-231118ossnewsl etterresend&utm_medium=email&utm_term=0_-5ebe84c9a8-%5BLI ST_EMAIL_ID%5D&mc_cid=f15e7d2ea1&mc_eid=518902b4bb

- **Helping Loved Ones Divided by Politics: Real People, Real Conversation:** Dr. Bill Doherty, a Marriage and Family Therapist and one of the founders of Braver Angels has videos of working with politically divided couples in therapy through the Center for Practice Transformation at the University of Minnesota. The following is a description of the training: "This session will focus on helping clients navigate the personal and relational minefields of political stress in their everyday lives. The presenter will use both his clinical experience and his leadership in Braver Angels, a national initiative to depolarize political 'reds' and 'blues,' and restore the fraying civic fabric." (Doherty, 2021).

Contact: This is a one hour video training for Mental Health Professionals available at: https://practicetransformation.umn.edu/continuing-educat ion/therapy-in-a-time-of-political-stress-and-polarization/

There are other examples of video sessions with Dr. Doherty available on YouTube at: www.youtube.com/results?search_query=bill+doherty+help ing+loved+ones+divided+by+politics

- **How Curiosity Will Save Us**: Mónica Guzmán is Senior Fellow for Public Practice at Braver Angels and host of A Braver Way, a podcast that equips people with the tools they need to bridge the political divide in their everyday lives. She is also the author of *I Never Thought Of It That Way: How to Have Fearlessly Curious Conversations in Dangerously Divided Times*. Both her podcast and YouTube talks are a good resource for clinicians, students and clients.

    Contact: YouTube talk: www.ted.com/talks/monica_guzman_how_curiosity_ will_save_us_jan_2022?utm_campaign=tedspread&utm_medium= referral&utm_source=tedcomshare

Support and Education:

- **Braver Angels Forum for Mental Health Professionals:** This is an on-line, monthly meeting for anyone in the mental health professions who is interested in a topic-focused, open discussion of how our field is being impacted by political issues. It is moderated by Paul Norris, LMFT (red) and Linda Chamberlain, PsyD (blue) and topics are suggested by the participants. Participants must register for the event in advance in order to receive any related materials that will be part of the discussion (e.g., videos, articles). It's an opportunity for us to share ideas, experiences, and perspectives about how politics and social issues are impacting us and our work in a respectful, supportive meeting.

    Contact: For more information: https://braverangels.org/event/forum-for-bra ver-angel-mental-health-professionals/2023-07-21/

- **Directory for Conservative Professionals:** This is a site for any mental health professionals who affirm conservative values. Professionals listed in the Directory "celebrate whatever Conservative political and religious values are important to you and your family … without you fearing that you will be judged, misunderstood, or controlled." Professional members of the Directory are committed to working with clients of various backgrounds, including clients who identify as liberal. This is a useful resource for clients who are seeking someone who aligns with conservative perspectives. Mental health professionals who register with the Directory can also access consultation and support with other members.

Contact: For more information: www.conservativeprofessionals.com/

INDEX

Note: Page numbers in **bold** refer to tables.

addictive behaviors 139–54; alcohol use 139, 141–2; cigarette smoking 139; conservative/liberal ideologies 140; funding 140; harm reduction approach 141; motivational interviewing 149–53; partisan sentiments 146–9; political biases 143–4; political differences 143–6; political spectrum 142–3; politics as stressor 141–2; recovery 142–3, 146–9, 153–4; self-help 153–4; social support 153–4; stigma 140; value-aligned counseling 149–53
advocacy 192–5
affective polarization 42, 83–5, 106
aggrieved entitlement 105
alcohol use 139, 141–2
American Counseling Association (ACA) 60, 196
American Mental Health Counselors Association (AMHCA) 196
American Psychiatric Association 34
American Psychological Association (APA) 60, 201
anger 126–9, 200–1
antipathy 46
antisocial personality disorder (ASPD) 123–4
appreciation 181–2
Attlee, Clement 35

authoritarianism **24**
autism spectrum disorder (ASD) 131–4
autonomy 12, 55, 86, 96–8, 149–51, 171, 187, 188, 190, 192, 195

beneficence 12, 187, 190, 195
Better Help™ 54, 62
bias: cognitive 17; confirmation 17, 41; depolarization 177–8; implicit 16; personal political 57–61; political 143–4
bipolar disorder 129–31
bipolar II disorder 129–31
Black Lives Matter movement 38, 46, 77
blank slate 77, 177, 194
borderline personality disorder (BPD) 6, 117–20
boundary management 190
boundary settings 166–7
Brexit 19, 26, 33, 38
Brown, Cheryl Dolinger 178
Butler, Judith 105

Canadian conservatism 39
cancel culture 22
Cattell, Raymond 15
Center for Disease Control (CDC) 201
Change Research survey 157
chronic stress 75–6

citizen therapist 13, 198–202; as
advocate role 199; anger reduction
200–1; as educator role 199; hostility
200–1; knowledge and skills 199;
mental health professionals 198;
misinformation 201–2; as organizers
199–200; perspectives 198–9
Civil Rights Act 34
Clean Air Act 35
client statements 10–11
clients *vs.* therapists 52–3
Clinton, Hillary 2
codependency 147
cognitive-behavioral therapy (CBT) 126,
128, 133
cognitive bias 17
cognitive dissonance theory 108–9
Cold War 36
collective trauma 105–8
communication skills 166, 179–81
communities of shared mourning 103
competence 190; cultural 190–1
confidentiality 190
confirmation bias 17, 41
conscientiousness **24**
conservative individuals 27
conservative therapists 51, 57, 62
cortisol 75
counseling 1–4, 8, 10–12, 20, 23, 25,
53, 60, 62, 69, 74; empathy 83–99;
individual partisanship model 44–7;
value-aligned counseling 149–53
countertransference 135
COVID-19 pandemic 23, 38–40, 50, 78,
97, 201
criterial referents 28
cultural competence 190–1
curricula 192–3

dating 156–8
dehumanization 41
depolarization 173–83; appreciation and
respect 181–2; biases, understanding/
acknowledging 177–8; communication
skills 179–81; information/training/
support 182–3; LAPP (listen/
acknowledge/pivot/perspective) skills
180–1; meaning of 173–4; political
divide 173–7; radical curiosity 178–9;
respect *vs.* cooperation 174–5
dialectical behavior therapy (DBT) 120
dialogue agents 30

differentiation 167–70
disappointment 126–9
discordant knowing 10
disenfranchised grief 111–2
divisiveness 1
Doherty, William 198
dopamine 25

economic axis 26
ego justification 42–3
emotions 41
empathy 83–99; affective polarization
83–5; critical attitudes 93; mental
health professionals 86–90, 93, 98;
neutrality 92–7, 99; partisan clients
83–5, 92–7; politically progressive
clients 87–8; political partisans 87–92;
politicized client goals 85–7; therapy
space 86, 89–91, 95–6
Environmental Protection Agency (EPA) 35
epigenetics 25
Equal Rights Amendment for women 35
ethical codes 12, 187
"The Ethical Lives of Clients:
Transcending Self-Interest in
Psychotherapy" (Doherty) 198
ethical practices 189–92; boundary
management 190; competence
190; confidentiality 190; cultural
competence 190–1; informed consent
190; professional integrity 191; social
responsibility 192
ethical principles: autonomy 12, 187, 188,
190, 192, 195; beneficence 12, 187,
190, 195; fidelity 12, 187, 189, 195;
justice 12, 187–9, 195; non-maleficence
12, 187, 190, 195
excessive subjective certainty *see* felt
knowledge
extended family 163
Eysenck, Hans 27

Falkland War 36
false consensus effect 7–11
families *see* relationships and families
felt knowledge 10
fidelity 12, 187, 189, 195
fight/flight response 75

Great Recession 37
grief 12, 102–14; collective trauma 105–8;
definition of 102; disenfranchised

111–2; mental health professionals 112–3; misused 103–5; nature of 102–3; partisan-related grief 109; personal identity 102; stages-of-grief model 103; tribalism as source 108–11; unresolved 113
group justification 43
Guralnik, Orna 159
Guzman, Monica 178

Haidt, Jonathan 28, 53
Haidt's theory 28–9
Hari, Johann 153
harm reduction approach 141
Harper, Stephen 40
Hillman, James 196
Hippocratic Oath 189
histrionic personality disorder (HPD) 121–3
Hoffer, Eric 9
hookup culture 157
hostility 200–1
hyper-partisanship 30, 127–9, 135

identity politics 29, 63
ideological group think 106
ideological polarization 42
implicit biases 16
implicit models 16–7
individual differences/personal preferences 43
individual liberties **21**
individual partisanship model 44–7
informed consent 190
ingroup/outgroup dichotomy 17
interpersonal family systems 164
intersectionality 193
"In the Year 2889" (Verne) 40
I statements 180

justice 12, 187–9, 195

Kant, Immanuel 188
Kathryn, Monica 173
Kerlinger's theory 28
Klein, Ezra 33, 176

LAPP (listen/acknowledge/pivot/perspective) skills 180–1
liberal bias 49–65
liberal/conservative differences models 15–31; addictive behaviors 140; attitudes with **21**; beyond axis 26–7;

implicit models 16–7; multifactor model, moral values 27–9; partisan identity model 29–30; psychological differences 23–6, **24**; science and differences 19–22; spectrum approach 17–9; "us-against-them" mentality 16–7
liberal therapists 3, 51, 52, 62, 63, 79, 144, 166, 195
licensed marriage and family therapists (LMFTs) 195
licensed professional counselors (LPCs) 195
Lincoln, Abraham 175
listening 180
logical learning theory 9

male patriarchy 60
marriage and family therapist (MFT) 52
mass political polarization 42
mental health conditions 116–36; anger, disappointment, and shame 126–9; antisocial personality disorder 123–4; autism spectrum disorder (ASD) 131–4; bipolar disorder 129–31; borderline personality disorder 117–20; histrionic personality disorder 121–3; misdiagnosis consequences 134–6; narcissistic personality disorder 120–1; paranoia 125–6; paranoid personality disorder 125–6
mental health practitioners 83, 192, 195, 203
mental health professionals 2–3, 7–8, 12–3, 41–2; advocacy 192–5; citizen therapist 198; clients *vs.* therapists 52–3; depolarization training 177–83; empathic neutrality 86–90, 93, 98; families 156, 158, 170–1; grief 112–3; liberal bias 49–65; neutrality 54–7; personal political bias 57–61; political divide 61–5; political mismatch 52–3; red flags 197; relationships 156, 158, 170–1; therapy space 70, 72, 74, 77–80
mental health services 49–52
misinformation identification 201–2
misused grief 103–5
morality **21**
motivational interviewing (MI) 149–53
multifactor model, moral values 27–9

narcissistic personality disorder (NPD) 120–1
National Association of Social Workers (NASW) 60, 196

National Health Service 35
National Organization for Human
    Services (NOHS) 196
neurotransmitters 25–6
Nixon, Richard 20, 35
non-maleficence 12, 187, 190, 195
noradrenaline 25
norepinephrine 25
normal distribution framework 18
Norris, Paul 64

online dating 157–8
openness **24**
Open Therapy Institute (OTI) 62
oppressors 60, 63

paranoia 125–6
paranoid personality disorder (PPD)
    125–6
parent-child relationship 160–1
partisan clients 83–5, 92–7
partisan identity 9; formation process
    41–2; model 29–30
partisan mindsets 7–11
partisan politicization 33–48; conservative
    politics 36–40; cultural divide 35–6;
    individual partisanship model 44–7;
    partisan identity formation process
    41–2; polarization spectrum 42–4;
    political divide 34–5; political
    divisiveness 33–4; single-issue politics
    36, 40
partisan-related grief 109
partisan sentiments 146–9
partisan sorting 29
past *vs.* optimism 27
perceived threats **24**
personal identity 4–7, 41; grief 102
personal political bias 57–61
perspective statements 181
pivoting 180–1
polarization spectrum 42–4
political affiliation 4–5
political bias 143–4
Political Compass model 26
political divide 12
political divisiveness 1, 12, 33–4, 47
political engagement 135
political extremism 87, 103, 135, 147–8
political identity 4–7, 111
political Manichaeism 75
political motivation 29

political orientations 17–8, 26, 30, 56,
    92–3
political partisans 19, 87–92
political polarization 5
political sentiment 17–8
political similarity 158–60
political spectrum 142–3
political stress 72, 75–6
political tribalism 110–1
political worldview 5
politicized families 168–70
politics gene 25
professional integrity 191
Progressive Conservative Party 39–40
progressive therapists 51, 63
psychodynamic splitting 6
psychological tribalism 29
public trust 197–8

"Q" phenomena 46

racism 75
radical curiosity 178–9
radical individuals 27
radicalism *vs.* conservatism 27
Reaganomics 35
Reagan, Ronald 35
recovery 142–3, 146–9, 153–4
red herring 72
relationships and families 156–71;
    boundary settings 166–7; dating 156–8;
    differentiation 167–70; extended family
    163; families as complex systems
    164–6; interpersonal family systems
    164; mental health professionals
    156, 158, 170–1; parent/child 160–1;
    political partisanship 164–6, 169;
    political similarity 158–60; politicized
    families 168–70; relentless hope 161;
    siblings 162–3; suggestions 170–1;
    Western model 156–7
relentless hope 161
respect 181–2
Rokeach, Milton 28

Safer, Jeanne 159
Schulz, Kathryn 173
self-help 153–4
self-identified liberals 4
self-interest **21**, 22
self in therapy 186
shame 126–9, 149

sibling relationships 162–3
single-issue politics 36, 40
smoking, cigarette 139
social axis 26
social cohesion **21**
social identity 5
social psychological effect 7
social responsibility 192
social support 153–4
spectrum approach 17–9
stages-of-grief model 103
stereotyping 186
stigma 140
stress: in addictive behaviors 141–2;
    chronic 75–6; hormones 75; political
    72, 75–6
substance abuse 140, 144–6, 148

tender-minded individuals 27
Thatcherism 35–6
Thatcher, Margaret 35
therapeutic alliance 2, 3, 51, 59, 69–70,
    77, 80, 85, 92, 97, 117, 144, 152, 171,
    182, 190
therapists 54–7; clients vs. 52–3;
    conservative 51, 57, 62; liberal 51, 62,
    63; political divide 61–5; progressive
    51, 63
therapy space 2, 11, 68–80; case study
    78–9; definition of 69; emotional
    well-being 79–80; empathic neutrality

86, 89–91, 95–6; mental health
    professionals 70, 72, 74, 77–80;
    political stress 72, 75–6; politics 71–5,
    77–8; uses of 70
tough-minded individuals 27
tough vs. tendermindedness 27
toxically partisanship 46, 85
tribalism 29–30; as grief source 108–11;
    political 110–1; psychological 29
Trump, Donald 2, 46, 77
trust: vs. distrust 27; public 197–8
two-axis model 27

ultimate attribution error 43
unresolved grief 113
"us-against-them" mentality 16–7, 41, 103

value-aligned counseling (VAC) 149–53
Ventura, Michael 196
Verne, Jules 40
Vietnam War 34
virtue-signaling 58
Voting Rights Act 34

Western relationship models 156–7
"We've Had a Hundred Years of
    Psychotherapy—and the World's
    Getting Worse" (Hillman and Ventura)
    196
"Why We're Polarized" (Klein) 33, 176
Women's Liberation Movement 34